Praise for Lisa Tillinger Johansen's
FAST FOOD VINDICATION

"Thoroughly researched... A cogent examination of the positive side of fast food, presented in a fresh, clear style."

-*Kirkus Reviews*

"As a dietitian, Lisa Tillinger Johansen knows what she is talking about! *Fast Food Vindication* is as important for people to understand as an urban survival guide."

-*Pacific Book Review*

"Astonishing. An enlightening read. I highly recommend this book for those on both sides of the fast food argument."

-*IP Book Reviewers*

I0026542

LISA TILLINGER JOHANSEN

STOP THE DIET, I WANT TO GET OFF!

Lisa Tillinger Johansen, MS, RD

J. Murray Press
Los Angeles, California
Cover design by Fishbrain
ISBN: 0996310207
ISBN 13: 9780996310208
Library of Congress Control Number: 20015906944

For Hiro, Jane, Gilbert, Mary, Lucille, Amelia, Jennie, Josie, Eduardo, Rosalba, Melida, Irene, Liz, Michael, John, and the rest of the Be Well gang. It's been an absolute pleasure.

CONTENTS

ACKNOWLEDGMENTS

Many thanks are due to those who were so generous with their time and observations.

Mike Tunison was my editor extraordinaire, and his guidance and good humor were invaluable to me and this book. Thanks also to Dana Moreshead from Fishbrain for wrapping it all up in a beautiful package with his striking cover design. And finally, to my beloved husband Roy, who believed in this book from the beginning and helped me across the finish line.

PART ONE

THE SKINNY

LISA TILLINGER JOHANSEN

INTRODUCTION

"The food here is terrible…And the portions are so small!"

—Writer/director Woody Allen

The idea for this book began at a wedding.

Who doesn't love a good wedding? The clothes, the flowers, the romance, the food…

Ah, the food. As we moved into the banquet hall for the reception, the culinary feast was on everyone's minds. It was all anyone seemed talk about. But for some reason, guests weren't conversing about the dishes being served; they were swapping stories of diets they had heard about from friends, magazine articles, even celebrities on talk shows.

I'm a registered dietitian with a master's degree in nutritional science and years of clinical and health education experience. I've counseled thousands of patients and clients on all of these diets. But hearing the guests only momentarily distracted me from my horrible faux pas of wearing white (gasp!) to a friend's wedding.

"I'm on the Blood Type Diet," said a woman with an impossibly high bouffant hairdo. "You've heard of that, haven't you? It's the one where you choose your foods based on your blood type. I'm an AB, so I'll be having the fish."

"Really?" her friend replied. "I *swear* by the gluten-free diet. I'm on it, my daughter's on it, and my granddaughter's on it."

I happened to know her granddaughter was six and didn't have a gluten sensitivity or celiac disease.

Then there was the stocky guy who was trying to impress one of the bridesmaids. "I'm a paleo man myself," he said, piling his plate high with beef kebabs. "It gives me more stamina, know what I mean? It puts me in touch with my inner caveman. There's a restaurant near my apartment that's paleo friendly. Maybe we can grab a bite there sometime, or…Hey wait, where are you going?"

And there were three Weight Watchers sisters who typed furiously on their phones and argued over their meals' point values. Apparently there was some discrepancy between their various apps, and the sisters' discussion was becoming more heated by the moment.

I'm past the point of being surprised by the wide range of weight-loss strategies—some worthless, some crazy, some quite reasonable—being tossed around. In the last few years, there has been a tidal wave of diets washing up on the shores of our nutritional consciousness. Celebrities prance across our screens, promoting a variety of weight-loss schemes on talk shows and infomercials. Medical doctors star in their own syndicated television programs, exposing millions to weight-management techniques, often unsupported by medical research. Other diets get traction on the Internet, racing all over the globe in social media posts, YouTube videos, and often unwanted spam e-mails. And it's hard to walk past a shopping center vitamin store without being approached by salespeople trying to pitch the latest weight-loss supplements. It seems that everyone wants a piece of the pie; the American diet industry tops $60 billion annually.

It's classic information overload. You can't blame people for being confused by all the diets out there, even as crazy as some of them may sound. I didn't speak up to my fellow wedding guests that day, but it occurred to me they would benefit from science-based facts about the diets they so ardently follow.

So during the toasts, I thought to myself, *I should write a book.*

I counsel clients on these matters each week, giving them information they need to make the best choices for their health and waistlines. I find that all too often there are issues with the diets presented to me in my counseling sessions and classes. They just plain don't work, particularly over the long term. And some of them are harmful, even potentially lethal. But it's also unhealthy to carry extra weight on our frames. So how do we separate good diets from the bad?

In the chapters to come, we'll take a good, hard look at the various weight-loss plans out there. I'll pull no punches in my professional evaluation of some of the most wildly popular diets, both bad and good, of the past few years. And along the way, I'll explore tried-and-true strategies for losing weight, based on my years of hospital experience, weight-loss seminars, and community outreach efforts. More often than not, the best answer is not a trendy celebrity-endorsed diet, but instead a few easy-to-follow guidelines that I've seen work in literally thousands of cases.

Enough is enough. It's time for the madness—and the diets—to stop.

ONE

Dieting…Who Hasn't?

"I feel like banging my head against the wall when I am asked what I think about the HCG Diet, Grapefruit Diet, or the Atkins Diet. Have we become so naïve as to believe that taking some homeopathic HCG drops will fix 20 years of poor eating? The sales say we have."

—Josh Hodnik, staff writer for VPX sports and *Muscle Evolution*

Holy cow, I'm fat! I've turned into a completely out-of-shape blob. I'm standing here looking in the mirror, and some stranger is staring back at me. Surely that's not me. Maybe if I put my glasses on…No, I'm still the same tub of lard. Bummer.

I don't know how this happened, or maybe I do a little

bit. But it just doesn't seem possible. I feel like just yesterday I was slim and trim, but now I can't button my pants. Aha, now I know why I've become so fond of stretch pants, baggy shirts, and sweaters…and Spanx.

This weight crept up on me, and now no matter what I do I can't get rid of it. I don't feel good about myself or like the way I look. And I think my health may be suffering because of it. I'm so depressed. I think I'm just going to go eat cake.

Sound familiar? Could that be you talking? If it is, join the club. A club, by the way, with many members. It's ever expanding. For some of us, this may be a scary first experience. You've been at a healthy weight all of your life…until now. Or you've had to watch what you eat, but still managed to maintain a comfortable weight. For others, this isn't your first go-round with this type of self-talk. There are many of us who've been up and down this path more than once. You might be in that vicious circle we like to call "yo-yo" dieting (a dieter's carousel, if you will)—repeated weight loss through dieting followed by a regain of the pounds lost. A 2012 study found the following:

- *26 percent of dieters in the United States adhered to their diets for less than a month*

- *36 percent followed theirs for a period of one to six months*

- *11 percent stuck to their diets for seven months to a year*

- *Only 27 percent stayed the course on their diet plans for over a year*

And it's not a surprise that almost 40 percent of Americans make their New Year's resolution about weight. And it's not shocking that only 8 percent keep it.

Weighty Matters

Dieting. It's almost easier to count those who *haven't* been on a weight-loss regimen sometime in their life than those who have. Have you ever gone on a diet? How about two, three, four, five, or more? I know that more than a few of you are nodding your heads vigorously. Or perhaps you're shaking your head in frustration. Don't worry, you're not alone.

The word *diet* means more than just what we do to lose weight. It also refers to what we eat and drink every day. It includes a prescribed diet, such as what a doctor or dietitian recommends for someone with, for example, diabetes or hypertension. We'll talk about all of these definitions in this book.

Just because I'm a dietitian doesn't mean I'm not human. I come from a family where many of us struggle to maintain a healthy weight. It definitely takes work for me to do so. And as I've aged, it has become harder. If I'm not diligent, I seem to expand almost overnight.

So, I'm in the weight management game with all of you. I know how you feel and the questions, challenges, and concerns you face. And with a master's degree in nutritional science and my licensure and experience as a registered dietitian, I know what works. I can help you.

Recently I had quite the unpleasant shock. I have a doctor's scale at home. The weights weren't set correctly, and I thought I weighed seven pounds less than I actually did. Ouch! I knew my clothes were a bit snug, but I'd chalked it up to a combination of temporary bloating and shrinking clothes. If only...

Weight-loss plans and diet products are a huge business in the United States. In 2012, Americans spent approximately $60 billion in their quest to lose pounds. Yes, you read it correctly. We spend a lot of dough in our effort to avoid being doughy. And over half of Americans (63 percent of females and 48 percent of males) would rather lose $1,000 of their own money than gain twenty pounds.

The desire to lose pounds and maintain a healthy weight isn't a bad idea. In fact, it's a really good one. But we don't always choose the best route to achieve this often elusive goal. Consequently, many of us are unsuccessful in our weight-loss attempts. Let's look at some statistics:

- *Three in ten Americans (25 percent of males and 32 percent of females) are currently trying to lose weight. About 55 percent of males have attempted to lose weight an average of four times each, while 73 percent of females have tried to shed pounds on average around seven separate times.*

- *A 2011 Gallup poll reported that about 52 percent of all US adults were successful at losing weight sometime in their life.*

- *In Britain, the average forty-five-year-old has already been on sixty-one diets.*

- *And while 62 percent of Canadians in one survey reported losing five or more pounds over a five-year period, most didn't maintain it; 70 percent of those who were overweight or obese gained back all, or sometimes more, of the pounds they shed after their initial weight loss.*

So many of us go round and round on the diet wheel. Do you remember when you weren't on a diet? Has it become a way of life for you? And how many different diets have you tried? Are you already looking for the next new thing? Perhaps you're one of the 35 percent of "occasional dieters" who move on to what's been termed "pathological dieting," or disordered eating. If that's you, aren't you tired of it?

There are certainly good reasons to lose weight. Carrying too much weight on our frames isn't healthy, but that's not stopping a lot of us from packing on the pounds. Obesity is also a negative trend we're seeing around the globe. The highest rates are in Oceania and the Middle East. Oh, and in the United States two-thirds of us are overweight or obese. It's a very dubious distinction. Here are the top-ten heaviest countries in the world, based on their 2013 overweight and obesity rates:

#1 American Samoa (94 percent)

#2 Kiribati, Central Pacific (82 percent)

#3 French Polynesia (74 percent)

#4 Saudi Arabia (73 percent)

#5 Panama (67.4 percent)

#6 United States (66.9 percent)

#7 Germany (66.5 percent)

#8 Egypt (66 percent)

#9 Kuwait (64 percent)

#10 Bosnia and Herzegovina (63 percent)

Kudos to the eight countries in Asia that have the lowest worldwide obesity rates. They are Vietnam, Laos, Indonesia, China, Japan, South Korea, the Philippines, and Singapore.

The obesity epidemic is a problem that must be dealt with. In 2013, the American Medical Association (AMA) took a major step by labeling obesity as a disease. While this brought on some controversy, it should result in a change in how health care providers look at and treat obesity in individuals. That's a good thing.

Fad or Fallacy

Carrying extra body weight can be quite bad for our health. It puts us at risk for a variety of diseases such as prediabetes, diabetes, hypertension, high cholesterol, joint problems, heart disease, sleep apnea, certain cancers, and more. Who wants that?

So what do so many of us do to combat our expanding girths? We go on a diet, often one that would be termed a "fad" diet. And we've been doing this for a lot longer than you might think.

Fad diets go back to at least 1087 when William the Conqueror came up with the alcohol-only diet. What was he thinking? Maybe he was too drunk to construct a more balanced one. Not surprisingly, this diet didn't work out for William. He died a year later after actually gaining weight.

The fad diet as we know it today arrived on the scene in the nineteenth century, when Sylvester Graham came up with the Graham diet. It focused on caffeine-free beverages and vegetarian meals. Not a bad idea, but it gets a bit weird. Part of the diet actually included eating graham crackers (go figure), as not only a way to assist in weight loss, but also to inhibit masturbation and the supposed blindness it caused. I'm not making this up.

In 1876, Englishman William Banting introduced the low-carbohydrate diet. A lot of us are familiar with this one. He lost fifty pounds with his plan and wrote the *Letter on Corpulence* discussing it. His weight-loss plan became so popular that in Britain the word *banting* became synonymous for dieting. A later version of this, the Atkins diet, would become very popular and is still being followed today.

Other early fad diets included Horace Fletcher's Great Masticator diet, which in 1903 suggested people chew their food thirty-two times. After doing this, they weren't to swallow it, but had to spit it out. That was certainly a low-calorie diet. And a lot of work for nothing.

The year 1928 gave us the Inuit diet, where followers could choose between eating either meat or the fat from it. Not both. There was also the bananas-and-skim-milk diet. And as recently as the late 1960s, Herman Taller, MD, advanced the "Calories Don't Count" diet. Before you embrace this concept, read on. It involved eating whatever you wanted and not worrying about quantity. The important aspect of this diet was that after you ate, you drank vegetable oil as a kind of chaser. Yuck. I'm sure that worked out well.

There are a lot of diets out there. Some are good. Many aren't. I'll talk about a lot of them throughout this book. I'll be your guide to choosing a healthy eating path and will give you the tools to navigate it. What I won't do is steer you toward a fad diet. In fact, I recommend you turn your back on them.

Fad diets are temporary and can be unhealthy. Very often they're restrictive. And many times they are, let's face it, a bit crazy.

People are drawn to fad diets because of the allure of quick results, which they sometimes deliver. But typically the weight loss can't be sustained long term. We're then faced with the disappointment and adverse health effects of reverting back to our prior weights. Or perhaps we may carry a heavier burden…on our bodies.

Close to 60 percent of adults in the United States want to shed at least twenty pounds.

It would be fantastic if we'd go to sleep one night and wake up the next day twenty pounds lighter. That's a good dream. But it's not realistic. So many of us want it to be true, and we try a lot of weight-loss programs with the hope that we'll be proven right. Optimism is high at the beginning. Some do have success that's maintained in the long term. Most don't.

Fad diets can be very difficult to adhere to for life. Even following them for months can be hard. We can also suffer ill effects from them such as headaches, nausea, constipation, diarrhea, nutritional deficiencies, hair loss, weakness, dizziness, fatigue, bad breath, loss of muscle, and more. Not fun.

Diets also affect the diseases we have. People with diabetes, kidney disease, and other conditions need to take care that these diets don't aggravate their conditions. More about health risks will be discussed in chapters to come.

Here's a crucial question: What's a fad diet? Some are easier than others to spot. Let's review some of their characteristics:

- *They promise a quick result.*
- *Statements are made about them that seem too good to be true or realistic.*
- *Simple conclusions are taken from involved studies.*
- *They take information from studies that haven't been peer reviewed. (Peer review and duplication of results is an important aspect of drawing reliable conclusions.)*
- *Statements of fact may be based on only one study. Again, results need to be tested and replicated to determine their quality.*
- *They rely on studies that don't have a large research group, or use those that look at only one segment of the population, such*

as African American males between the ages of thirty and forty-five or Caucasian women ages sixty-five to eighty.

- *Assertions are made that highly regarded medical- and science-based organizations refute.*
- *Their statements or recommendations are used to try to sell us their products.*
- *They promote "special elixir" type foods or specific food combinations.*
- *They suggest that food can affect body chemistry.*
- *Foods are identified as either "bad" or "good."*
- *They eliminate foods or food groups.*

Do any of these ring a bell? Have you researched or tried a diet with one or more of the above characteristics? Who's nodding? Here are some of the fad diets you might've explored:

3-Day diet

Apple-cider-vinegar diet

Atkins diet

Beverly Hills diet

Blood Type Diet

Cabbage-soup diet

Cleanses

Coconut-oil diet

Dukan diet

Grapefruit diet

hCG diet

Hollywood Diet

Paleo Diet

South Beach Diet

Zone Diet

My husband is on the brown diet. It's a simple one. If it's brown, he eats it. This isn't healthy, as it's filled with items like fried chicken, french fries, and pizza. He's getting better, though. I got him to get rid of the fryer he had in his bachelor days. But he's still a work in progress.

The online pharmacy UKMedix.com found that 71 percent of women had tried a fad diet. Here's the breakdown of the diets they tried:

Laxatives: 47 percent

Fasting: 45 percent

Cabbage soup diet: 39 percent

Liquid diet: 35 percent

Body wraps: 29 percent

Cereal diet: 26 percent

Baby food diet: 26 percent

Raw food diet: 24 percent

Small plates: 18 percent

Eating foods known to make you sick: 14 percent

I question more than a few of these diets. Do you? If not, you should.

It's Not a Clique, It's a Group

Restrictive, low-calorie, and other types of fad diets aren't only challenging to follow, they can also be nutritionally unbalanced. For example, cutting out entire food groups or a significant portion of them may result in not getting adequate calories, vitamins, minerals, and more. Or we may get an overabundance of something. This can cause health issues for some, like potential kidney problems from excessive protein. Too little or too much of something isn't a good thing. Our bodies like balance.

Protein, fruits, vegetables, grains, dairy, and healthy fats should all have a place in our diets. Our bodies use all of these for a variety of things. Making the more nutritious choices out of these groups is, of course, important. And each of them does have healthy members. When we cut out a food group or a significant part of it, we're short-changing ourselves. We'll talk more about the food groups later on.

Knowledge Is Power

Another key component of weight loss and maintenance is gaining the tools we need to manage our eating for life. It requires knowledge and behavior change. The former isn't likely difficult for most of us, although there are a lot of less credible sources out there. The latter can be a seemingly impossible task. This book will help you tackle both.

We're so lucky to live in a day and age in which books, magazines, journals, newspapers, websites, blogs, and more are so readily available and abundant. The Internet has expanded our horizons and our learning ability to such an amazing degree. Practically any information we want or need is just a keystroke away. But we must make sure that what we're reading, even relying on, is quality and expert.

When I first went to college back in the day, personal computers didn't exist. I know, can you imagine? All research had to be done at the library. And we had to use card catalogues to find our material. It was slow going.

I've thought about this often while writing my books.

It's certainly quick to tap into my own knowledge, which I do extensively. But when I want to look something up, I'm happy that it's easy and convenient to find.

When looking for nutrition information on the web, I recommend perusing the sites that you know are science-based. Medical and government websites such as mayoclinic.com and cdc.gov are reputable. So are sites like eatright.org and choosemyplate.gov. You can also go to registered dietitian sites like mine at consultthedietitian.com. You have a question? I'll answer it. For other online sources, please review the Appendix for more sites that I like and trust.

Experts in the field can be great sources. Registered dietitians are a fantastic go-to for information about nutrition. But there are so many other people out there, including celebrities, who have their own diet plans or champion them. It's important to note that these people often don't have the training necessary to assess and recommend an appropriate diet plan. Tread lightly there. Designations like RD, RDN, RN, and MD signify experts in health care, including diet and nutrition.

In Britain, 47 percent of people who are watching their weight will try a diet because a celebrity is on it.

I counsel many people each year regarding a variety of health issues, including weight management, prediabetes, diabetes, high cholesterol, hypertension, heart disease, kidney disease, malnutrition, and more. Many of them are well-versed in self-care and have solid facts and plans to achieve and maintain good health. Others could use some help.

Television shows, magazines, books, our families, friends, neighbors, coworkers, personal trainers, vitamin store personnel, and others often share advice. Many of us take that and run with it. Sometimes we shouldn't.

It's essential that we use a filter and common sense when sorting through the barrage of information that comes our way. If it sounds too good to be true, it most likely is. The promise of five pounds of weight loss in several days or ten pounds in one week, for example, isn't healthy or advisable. It's tempting, I know. But in this case, slow and steady wins the race.

What do you need to get started on a healthy eating plan for you? A great beginning is to understand the pros and cons of all the major diet plans out there. Having reliable facts and figures, determining your desire and willingness to change, and setting some goals are important. Knowing recommended portion sizes and the balance of the food groups is essential. The contribution of physical activity and the effectiveness of using measuring and benchmark tools help round out a powerful weight-management arsenal. I can help you with all of these, and there's no time like the present. It's time to stop the diet and get on with a long-term eating plan for life.

So let's get off the dieting merry-go-round. Our healthy weight lies ahead.

LISA TILLINGER JOHANSEN

TWO

Why?

"It's the same old line that we have always been told—we too could be thinner, younger, or more loved, if we would only buy whatever new, improved diet food or regimen is on offer. And we still fall for it."

—Louise Foxcroft, author of *Calories & Corsets*

Why do we do it? What makes us try the latest and greatest fad diet, or go back in time for an oldie, but not so goodie? For many, it's the quick fix. We want fast results, sometimes for an upcoming special event, or as a jump start for a long-term plan. We're impatient and don't want to wait. We have to have it *now* and fad diets are alluring for this very reason.

Vanity, too, plays a role here. We want to change the way we look, often as fast as we can, and that's very motivating. It can influence us to choose weight and inches over health.

A small study found that 75 percent of participants would take a pill that would guarantee they would reach or maintain their preferred weight even if it reduced their life expectancy. In fact, they'd throw away on average 5.7 years. Almost all in the study, 91 percent, wouldn't take a pill that would increase their lifespan by five years if it meant they'd stay overweight. That's mind boggling to me. And it's ironic, since healthy eating and exercise may help us lose weight and live longer. That's more bang for your buck.

Some brides-to-be have prepared for their upcoming nuptials with the feeding-tube diet, aka the K-E diet. They literally get fed a low-calorie diet via a feeding tube that's inserted through the nose, down the esophagus, and into the stomach. They do this willingly for quick weight loss.

Tube feeding is the manner in which people are provided nutrition who can't or won't eat on their own. It shouldn't be used as a dieting method to fit into a wedding dress, or as anything else for that matter.

Carrying too much weight on our frames can affect more than our health. Researchers at Yale University found that weight discrimination has increased greatly in the United States, to the point that it's as prevalent as reported cases of racial discrimination. It especially impacts women. This bias leads to unequal treatment in health care, employment, and education. There have even been cases where some women have been chastised while eating in public. Overweight and obese women are not as likely to marry or be hired for a job, and are typically paid less. This is a sad state of affairs.

Overweight and obese people are often unfairly stereotyped. Some see them as lacking self-discipline and they question their competence. They're labeled as sloppy, lazy, and unmotivated. This can be hurtful and unfair. It might drive someone to look for a quick path to a thinner body.

Hear No Evil, See No Evil...Right?

There's another reason why we try fad diets. And it's a big one—advertising. Catchy commercials, hum-worthy jingles, and believable testimonies bombard us constantly via all forms of media. And they transfix us because marketing and advertising firms know how to reach us.

- *Our emotions play a big part in our purchasing decisions. We rely on our feelings and experiences when making choices over facts and brand attributes.*

- *Our intent to buy an advertised product is far more influenced by our emotional response to the ad rather than the actual content of the advertisement itself (two-to-one for print ads and three-to-one for TV commercials). Studies conducted by the Advertising Research Foundation concluded that the emotion of "likeability" is the measure most predictive of whether an advertisement will increase a brand's sales.*

- *Researchers have found that positive emotions toward a brand are a bigger influence on consumer loyalty than brand attributes and trust.*

- *Emotions are the main reason we like brand name products.*

- *And let's face it. Our weights, our looks, and our health can be very emotional for us.*

Weight-loss products and diets are big business. And through marketing and advertising we're constantly being bombarded with attempts to get us to try them. In addition to health, romance, happiness, nostalgia, family, hot bods, and the like, what else really helps draw us in? It's none other than the celebrity spokesperson and advocate. And it may not matter if the diets they tout are healthy or make sense. Lisa Dorfman, RD, and spokesperson for the American Diabetic Association sums up the psychology of many who follow a celebrity-endorsed fad diet: "They just like the way she looks and they'd like to look like her, too." So let's talk about Tinsel Town.

Lights, Camera...Diet

Oh, that crazy Hollywood. What those celebs won't try in their quests to maintain those incredibly thin bodies. And, believe me, if you haven't seen an actor or actress in real life, many of them are much smaller than you might imagine. Remember, it's said that the camera puts on ten pounds. And it really appears to do just that.

I once saw an actress, who will remain unnamed, while I was in the studio audience of a talk show. She walked out on the stage resplendent in beautiful clothes, with her hair and makeup perfectly done. She looked fantastic. But when she turned to go sit down next to the host, I lost sight of most of her. I'm not kidding. I saw a head and hair and that's about it. Imagine a floating head and you get the picture. You know, the lollipop shape. Her body frame was so slim it practically disappeared from view when she turned sideways. Not good.

Perhaps some of you are saying, hey, that sounds awesome to me. But you must ask yourself this question: Can you be too thin? Please put your hands on the side of your heads and stop the horizontal movement. The answer is a vertical nod. It's yes. Being underweight can cause nutritional deficiencies. Do you want that? Now you can let your head take a horizontal turn.

The reality is that it's hard for so many of us just to get to and maintain a healthy weight. And sometimes our idea of what that is gets skewed. Much of the public's fascination with underweight actors, musicians, models and other celebrities seen on TV, in movies, and in often air-brushed magazine spreads doesn't help. Too many of us go to great and unhealthy lengths to try for a weight and look that's impossible, as well as ill advised, to get.

Take the case of twenty-four-year-old Michele Kobke in Germany, who as of June 2013 had worn a corset 24/7 for three years. Her reason for doing this was to reduce the size of her waist. And she has. She started off at a waist circumference of twenty-five inches (already considered to be small and healthy) and got it down to an incredibly tiny sixteen-inch circumference. But she isn't satisfied. She'd like for her waist to reach fourteen inches. This would beat Cathie Jung's world record of smallest adult waist at fifteen inches. I was a wee babe when I last had a waist this small.

This extreme measure has affected Kobke's health. She has difficulty standing up without the corset because her stomach and back muscles are weak. Her balance has been compromised as well. She appears to have difficulty taking deep breaths, and in a recent ultrasound it was found her stomach has been pushed into an abnormal position.

Should she keep this up, what might happen to her? I shudder to think.

Some celebs have also turned to corsets. There's at least one known female who wore *two* corsets night and day for three months after giving birth. Who was it, you ask? Actress Jessica Alba. She did this in an attempt to help her quickly lose the weight she gained during pregnancy. How did it go for her? "It was sweaty, but it was worth it," she reported. "It was brutal; it's not for everyone." The corset diet appears to have gained a few more celebrity followers, including TV reality star Kim Kardashian and former real housewife of Atlanta Kim Zolciak.

Beauty pageant contestants can also overdo it. Kirsten Haglund, Miss America 2008 said about the 2013 competition: "The girls, I thought, were much too thin. I agree that if you would have tested their BMIs they probably would have been much too thin. And that's the standard in the modeling industry and the fashion industry as well."

From beauty pageants and on to the fashion industry, so many people are super thin. And more than a few go to restrictive lengths to achieve this thinness. I remember back during the pinnacle of Cindy Crawford's modeling career when she spoke about how she and three other supermodels would take a hamburger, cut it in fourths and each eat a piece for their meal. It was apparently a splurge for them.

Recently, allegedly unretouched pictures of Cindy Crawford from a December 2013 photo shoot for a magazine cover surfaced online. In the pictures, Crawford is wearing a bikini and you can see that while she's definitely thin, her midsection and thighs aren't as toned as they appeared to be when she was younger. Most people, including myself, thought she looked great. And given that she's still a model with a physique that many of us would be hard-pressed to achieve, the pictures of her body looked more like a true depiction of how a fit woman in her mid to late forties might look. A controversy exists, though, as the photographer who took the photos, as well as Crawford's husband, dispute that the pictures were the real thing. There was some suggestion that they were doctored to make Crawford look bad. Either way, I think she looks great.

I'm not sure there are a whole lot of magazine covers and ads that aren't altered in some way. We've all seen "before" and "after" pictures of well-known people, as well wondered what happened to an arm, leg, or blemish on a model or celebrity that is smaller or even missing in action in a photo spread. And who wouldn't mind seeing a few photos altered to make themselves look better. That's human, but it's a crazy practice. What so many people aspire to look like isn't even real. It's just editing.

One of my favorite Photoshop stories is from 2006, when a magazine cover of Katie Couric promoting her joining CBS Evening News was altered to make her look thinner. Apparently Couric was surprised by the edit, commenting, "I liked the first picture better because there's more of me to love." Good for her.

But the reality is there's a particular look some individuals want to portray and advertise. Using underweight models in advertising is commonplace. This is concerning because it can affect how all of us, including the normal folk, view our bodies, and that can impact our self-esteem. It can certainly impact our eating habits, often in a negative way.

There are tragic cases, including the case of twenty-one-year-old Brazilian model Ana Carolina Reston who died in 2006 of complications from anorexia nervosa. She sadly joined the growing list of other models who also succumbed to this disease.

But there may be change on the horizon. In late 2014, regulators forced Urban Outfitters Europe to remove a picture of a model from the United Kingdom website because she was thought to be too thin. The reason cited was "her inner thigh gap promoted an image that was irresponsible and harmful." That's a giant step in the right direction.

France just passed a law that would impose a six-month prison sentence for managers of modeling agencies that employ underweight models. It would also be a criminal offense to promote "excessive skinniness." The French want to stop sites encouraging eating disorders or promoting "pro-anorexia" and "thinspiration." Models on the catwalk must prove they have a healthy body mass index (BMI) per government standards. Israel, Spain, and Italy have similar laws. Wow.

While it may seem I'm celebrity-crazed, it's really just a normal, reasonable interest. Don't worry, celebs, I'm not stalking you. I bring them up because as famous people, they have voices that can be heard around the world. A lot of people watch them, listen to them, and aspire to be like them. Quite a few celebrities diet. And many of them talk about it. They can sway opinion and action with regard to what and how some of us eat or don't eat, and how we want to look and weigh. It's something to

think about.

Many actors, entertainers and models diet to get and keep work. And this has been true for quite a while. In the 1920s, Gayelord Hauser, a "diet guru" and Greta Garbo's romantic interested, proclaimed, "most of our high-priced movie stars are living in constant fear of losing their attractiveness and thereby their popularity…they simply can't afford to become fat and unattractive."

Members of both sexes certainly can feel the pressure to look and feel good about themselves. In some careers, and perhaps in life in general, some feel that women are held to a higher standard. I love the joke that host Tina Fey made during the 2015 Academy Awards when talking about the time it took for a male actor to be made-up as a character for a movie role. Fey quipped, "Steve Carell's makeup took two hours to put on, including his hairstyle and makeup. Just for comparison, it took me three hours today to prepare for my role as Human Woman." You gotta laugh.

Celebrity lives look wonderful and glamorous. They have fame and fortune. They're beautiful, handsome, and just look overall fantastic. Life seems easy for them. They appear to have it all, whether it's true or not. While that doesn't float everyone's boat, it does for so many.

What we tend to forget, though, is the amount of time, effort, money, surgery, styling and airbrushing that often goes into their look. We ignore the fact many celebs have a lot of help from personal chefs, fitness trainers, stylists, and more. More importantly, we often forget they're human. They're not perfect, and in the case of dieting, they're not usually experts.

Yet so many of us jump on their diet bandwagons without much thought. We put our health in their hands. And we shouldn't.

Certainly not considered to be diet experts, reality-show celebrities the Kardashian sisters (Kim, Kourtney, and Khloe) were paid endorsers for the weight-loss drug Quick Trim. And they ultimately became defendants in a 2012 five-million-dollar class action lawsuit, accused of making misleading and false claims about the product's results.

Even celebrities who people presume are experts have been questioned. In 2014, cardiothoracic surgeon and TV-show host Mehmet Oz, MD, was brought to task by the United States Congress for statements he made about weight-loss products on his program. While he was adamant about his belief in the products, he admitted, "I recognize they don't have the scientific muster to present as fact…"

In late 2014, the *British Medical Journal* took a look at two shows, *The Dr. Oz Show* and *The Doctors*. They sampled forty random episodes and reviewed 445 recommendations made on *The Doctors* and 479 recommendations on *The Dr. Oz Show*. They found that half of the claims made on these two programs didn't have any scientific basis and some even contradicted current scientific conclusions. Science educator

Samuel W. Bennett put together a great pictorial of their findings:

Television Doctor Recommendations: Dr. Oz and The Doctors

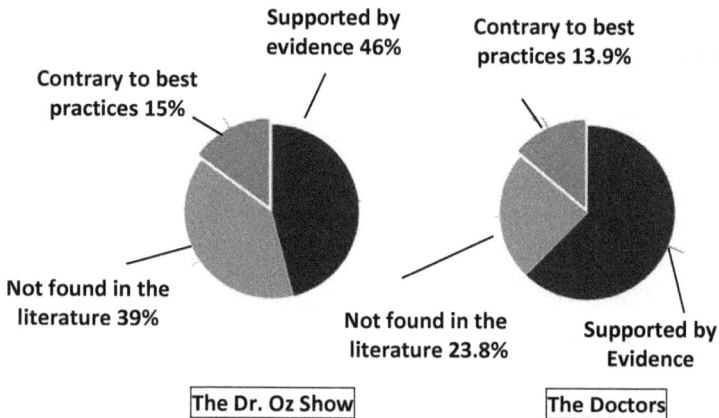

The Dr. Oz Show
- Supported by evidence 46%
- Contrary to best practices 15%
- Not found in the literature 39%

The Doctors
- Contrary to best practices 13.9%
- Not found in the literature 23.8%
- Supported by Evidence

That's a humble pie of statistics. And it's not surprising. I hear so many people quoting Dr. Oz, emphatically certain that whatever health-related tidbit he shared on his show is good for them to follow. He does dispense some good advice, but as the United States Congress found, not always.

It's also important to not overstate or make guarantees. Many of us grab on to that and don't want to let go. In 2015, Dr. Oz introduced a new magazine called *The Good Life*. A headline on the first cover reads, "DROP 10 POUNDS YOU WON'T GAIN BACK." How does he know we won't gain the weight back? That seems like a promise he likely can't keep.

This pattern of behavior has caused consternation among some in the medical community, including myself. In April 2015, ten doctors sent a letter to Columbia University's College of Physicians and Surgeons, where Dr. Oz is vice chair of the Department of Surgery, urging the university to cut ties with the celebrity doc. It was quite scathing. Here are some of the more salient complaints:

"Dr. Oz is guilty of either outrageous conflicts of interest or flawed judgments about what constitutes appropriate medical treatments, or both. Whatever the nature of his pathology, members of the public are being misled and endangered."

"He has repeatedly shown disdain for science and for evidence-based medicine..."

"...he has manifested an egregious lack of integrity by promoting quack treatments and cures in the interest of personal financial gain."

A short time later, five medical doctors and three PhDs from Columbia University penned an op-ed in *USA Today* about Dr. Oz. While they said that Dr. Oz shouldn't be terminated from a "well-earned position in academic medicine" at Columbia University, they also mentioned among other concerns: "Many of us are spending a significant amount of our clinical time debunking Ozisms regarding metabolism game changers."

That's got to hurt. But I know what they're talking about. I often have to debunk them as well.

Dr. Oz fought back in part by questioning the qualifications and integrity of some of the doctors who authored the first letter. He also stated that his show is not really a medical program. Dr. Oz told NBC's Matt Lauer, "We very purposely, on the logo, have 'Oz' as the middle, and the 'Doctor' is actually up in the little bar for a reason. I want folks to realize that I'm a doctor, and I'm coming into their lives to be supportive of them. But it's not a medical show."

And Columbia University released this statement: "Columbia is committed to the principle of academic freedom and to upholding faculty members' freedom of expression for statements they make in public discussion." Meanwhile, the AMA recently announced they're going to be more proactive in holding doctors in the media accountable for their words and actions.

20/20: Perfect Eyesight, not a Perfect Diet

Another celebrity healthcare professional, psychologist Phil McGraw, Ph.D, known for the *Dr. Phil* show often weighs in on dieting. In 2014 he wrote a book titled *The 20/20 Diet*. His plan prescribes its followers to eat twenty key ingredients or foods he says may increase our body's thermogenesis with the goal of speeding up metabolism and burning more calories.

Thermogenesis is the production of heat. Diet-induced thermogenesis refers to the increase in energy (calories) expended in metabolizing our food. Typically it's between 5 and 15 percent of our daily expended energy. Studies have shown that protein increases thermogenesis. Protein also makes us feel full, known as satiety. Dr. McGraw refers to this in his book.

There are three phases to his plan, culminating in a management phase. The first phase requires eating four daily meals that only include the twenty key foods. That's very limited. As you move through the phases, more foods can be added to the initial twenty allowed. Exercise and other positive behavior change are encouraged.

The book is difficult to read, and I find the diet confusing. It's also too structured and restrictive, particularly in the early phases. One enamored 20/20 diet follower wrote in a review, "no food eliminated, but simply put off." But temporary exclusion is still exclusion.

Dr. McGraw does provide some good advice. And he did work with a dietitian. But his 20/20 plan is packaged in the trappings of a fad diet. Balance and moderation, not questionable exclusions, is the better path.

When we follow a famous person, health care professional or not, down a crazy diet path, it can affect our health. Why do we place our trust in them? What makes them an expert? Does being famous mean they have all the diet answers? Why should we listen to them? After all, it's our health on the line. Our diets affect our bodies. Let's be smart here. I call "cut" on this scene.

LISA TILLINGER JOHANSEN

THREE

Gluten, We Hardly Knew Ye!

"Gwyneth Paltrow's 'Elimination Diet' Is Hardly the Craziest Diet to Come Out of Hollywood."

—Liat Kornowski, *Huffington Post*

Notwithstanding those who shouldn't diet because they're already at a healthy weight or are underweight, the reality is that many of us should shed some pounds. If we carry too much weight on our frames, we'll benefit from doing so. And, as already mentioned, a lot of us try some crazy things to do just that. One of them is cutting out or severely limiting certain foods or entire food groups from our diets.

They're called elimination diets. And they've morphed into something they weren't ever really meant to be. In fact, their original intention had nothing to do with weight loss. An elimination diet is used to determine what foods might be causing symptoms in those with food sensitivities.

The Science of Sensitivity

Recently, actress Gwyneth Paltrow coauthored a cookbook called *It's All Good*. A reviewer for the *Guardian* took a look at it. She felt that the book was more about "a complete fear of food" and cited Paltrow's inspiration for the book struck "when she nearly died after eating too many french fries." How many fries did that woman eat?

Anyway, Paltrow went to her doctor and was told her "body was in crisis," and that she was allergic to a lot of foods, including corn, peppers, and aubergine. That's a very unique combo.

Paltrow promotes the Clean 21-day elimination diet. Created by cardiologist and "cleanse specialist" Alejandro Junger, MD, it's designed to remove "all foods from our diet that are known to cause food allergies, food sensitivities, and cause disruptions in the digestive process." It excludes *a lot* of foods. Too many, and all at once.

The diet calls for liquids only at breakfast and dinner. Lunch consists of solids from the approved foods list. Twelve hours must pass between dinner and breakfast. For some, like diabetics (who shouldn't be on this diet anyway), that's too long to go without food.

Believe it or not, the key to success on this diet is... bowel movements. Really. And if you don't have one every day, you're encouraged to do a variety of things to rev up your colon, including using herbal laxatives, colonics and castor oil. I'm not a fan of this, or for that matter, any part of this diet.

As a celebrity, Paltrow is able to voice her opinions and experiences to the public at large. That's fine. But these may be unique to her and may not apply to most. I recommend evaluating your own particular symptoms and food intake with your health care provider in order to determine if there's a real need to eliminate certain foods from your diet.

Only 3 percent of people have a true food allergy.

Unless we have a food sensitivity or allergy, have triggers like spicy foods that may aggravate a condition like acid reflux, have diseases, or take medications that restrict certain items, it's typically not necessary to limit or avoid foods or food groups.

For those with food sensitivities, symptoms can be a real problem. They can interfere with quality of life, so it's important to find the cause. Take a look at some of the following signs and symptoms:

Irritability

Nasal congestion

Dark circles under eyes

Headache

Aching muscles

Abdominal pain

Fatigue

Hyperactivity

Attention deficit

Memory loss

I have to caution here that the above symptoms can be indicative of many diseases or conditions. Or their appearance may mean nothing major at all. If you're experiencing one, some, or all of these, I recommend seeing your doctor about it. If there's some underlying cause, it's important to make sure you get the correct diagnosis.

Sometimes it's challenging to figure out which foods are causing you problems. That's when an elimination diet comes in handy. Let's take a look at how it works:

1. *Before beginning a diet, keep a diary or symptom inventory for at least three days.*

2. Continue the symptom diary while you're following the diet.

3. To identify specific food sensitivities, eat one of the eliminated foods per day and note any reactions. Symptoms may occur within a few minutes, a few hours, or the next day.

4. Continue the diet for five to ten days, until there is convincing improvement in your symptoms lasting forty-eight hours.

5. Carry out the diet at an appropriate time. Don't try it during a holiday.

While I have no food sensitivities, I've experienced just about all of the symptoms that can be attributed to them at some point or another. And unfortunately for my husband, irritability and memory loss seem to be my main visitors right now. Hello, menopause...

It's Nothing to Sneeze At

While some of us have food sensitivities or autoimmune disorders affected by food, there are others who have food allergies. A food allergy is defined as "an immune system reaction that occurs soon after eating a certain food." Even a tiny amount of the allergy-causing item can trigger signs and symptoms such as digestive problems, hives, or swollen airways. In some people, a food allergy can cause severe symptoms or even a life-threatening reaction known as anaphylaxis. From gastrointestinal issues to death, they can be a pain in the butt. Literally. If you think you may have a food allergy, see your doctor about it. And it's certainly essential to avoid the foods in question and be prepared for treatment should you accidentally ingest the problematic item.

Common Food Allergies

Eggs
Shellfish
Fish
Tree nuts
Peanuts
Wheat
Milk

There are some of us who flirt with the thought that we're allergic to certain foods when we actually aren't. It can be frustrating to try to pinpoint the causes of the various symptoms that many of us live with, either now and then, or more frequently. But it's important that we don't develop an unhealthy or fearful relationship with food.

Gluten and the Gut

Gluten is a protein found in wheat, rye, barley, and

triticale (cross between rye and wheat). It provides elasticity to dough and helps it to rise. Gluten hardens during baking, which aids the item being prepared to maintain its shape. Many foods contain gluten. It can be found in bread, cereal, pasta, crackers, cookies, soy sauce, and beer.

There are some of us who have very real problems associated with gluten. People with celiac disease, an autoimmune disorder affected by ingesting this protein, are one such group. When someone with celiac disease eats food containing gluten, it causes their white blood cells, our body's army against its enemies, to go on the attack. This can cause damage to the intestinal wall. Consequently, it affects digestion and absorption of nutrients. The result can be abdominal pain, diarrhea, and mineral deficiencies.

Some of us have an intolerance to gluten, but don't have celiac disease. This is called nonceliac gluten sensitivity. Approximately 1 percent of the world's population has celiac disease. This includes about three million Americans. In Australia, while around one million of its residents have eliminated wheat from their diets, only one-quarter of them have done so because of a medical condition.

Many people without a health reason are currently on gluten-free diets. In fact, a recent poll found that 30 percent of adults either wanted to reduce gluten consumption or completely rid it from their diets. In 2010, *Time* put the gluten-free diet in the number-two spot on its list of top-ten food trends. This, of course, has been a boon to the gluten-free product industry. It's estimated that one out of five adult consumers currently purchases gluten-free foods.

Since 2008 the gluten-free product industry has grown 28 percent each year. According to Nielsen data, sales of gluten-free items in the United States totaled $19.7 billion for the year ending May 2013. This was more revenue than that derived from high-fiber, multigrain, or cholesterol-free items generated.

And let me tell you, some of these products can be quite costly. I recently threw a party and bought one bottle of gluten-free beer (two servings' worth) for my friend who has a sensitivity to gluten. It cost close to nine dollars! I was shocked. And I was further disappointed because she didn't drink it. But no worries. It still resides in my fridge, waiting for the time that she'll want to crack that brewski open.

Daniel A. Leffler, MD, director of clinical research at the Celiac Center at Boston's Beth Israel Deaconess Medical Center, feels my gluten-free sticker shock pain. "People who are sensitive to gluten may feel better, but a larger portion will derive no significant benefit from the practice," he says. "They'll simply waste their money, because the products are expensive." No kidding.

Two of the main reasons many of us embark on the gluten-free ride are the assertions that this diet can result in weight loss and more energy. It also doesn't hurt that a number of celebrities have followed it or still do, including Oprah Winfrey, Victoria Beckham, Gwyneth Paltrow, Lady Gaga, Miley Cyrus, and tennis star Novak Djokovic. But do the weight management and increased energy claims stand up to scrutiny? It depends on whom you ask.

Singer Miley Cyrus has gone on Twitter to deny the rumors that she has the eating disorder anorexia nervosa. She let her followers know she's allergic to lactose and gluten. "It's not about weight—it's about health. Gluten is crap anyway!" She went on to say, "Everyone should try no gluten for a week! The change in your skin, physical, and mental health is amazing. You won't go back!"

As I write this, Cyrus has more than nineteen million followers on Twitter. This story was also picked up by many media outlets, including *US* magazine, *People* magazine, *CBS News*, *Huffington Post*, Eonline, TODAY.com, and more. That creates a very large sphere of influence. And she's not the only celebrity to suggest a gluten-free diet. Kim Kardashian also got into the act by tweeting, "Gluten-free is the way to be." She has more than thirty-two million Twitter followers and gets a great deal of press, as you may have noticed.

With regard to weight loss, it's likely that gluten-free dieters shed pounds because by eliminating certain foods they also cut calories and less nutritious choices such as desserts. Anybody who reduces the amount of high-fat and high-calorie foods eaten may lose weight. It doesn't matter if the foods contain gluten or not. Gastroenterologist Mark DeMeo of Chicago's Rush University Medical Center agrees: "There's nothing magical about a gluten-free diet that's going to help you lose weight." Success on this diet largely depends on what the gluten-free foods are replaced with. It's all about calories in versus calories expended.

As far as an increase in energy, it can be argued that changing your diet to a healthy, balanced one will help with that. Losing weight can make us feel better, which can energize us. This can be accomplished whether we're gluten free or not.

In a recent interview about the gluten-free diet, Stefano Guandalini, MD, medical director of the Celiac Disease Center at the University of Chicago, said, "It is not a healthier diet for those who don't need it." He went on to say that those who do it for no medical reason "are following a fad, essentially," speculating that no more than 1 percent of people have gluten sensitivity.

There's a lack of scientific evidence suggesting that avoiding gluten results in weight loss. Many gluten-free products have the same amount of calories, or even more, than their gluten-containing counterparts. This may be due to the fact that sometimes gluten is replaced in products with flour that has added fat or sugar to make them tasty. This results in a higher-calorie product.

Dunkin' Donuts recently announced plans to sell gluten-free donuts. Interestingly, these items may have more calories than the ones with gluten. The wheat-free donut weighs in at 320 calories, while the glazed donut with gluten has 260 calories.

If we don't have celiac disease or gluten sensitivity, are there any beneficial health effects from going on a gluten-free diet? Studies have shown that there aren't. In fact, it might be detrimental. This is because gluten-free diets can be low in iron, folate, niacin, thiamin, calcium, phosphorus, zinc, vitamin B12, and fiber. We need all of these and throughout this book I'll cover many of the vitamins and minerals. Let's start with a few:

Folate (and folic acid)—*This water-soluble B vitamin is found in green leafy vegetables, cereals, orange and tomato juice, mushrooms, legumes, fruit (such as lemons, melons, and bananas), organ meats, asparagus, okra, and baked goods. It can help prevent neural-tube defects during pregnancy.*

Thiamin—*Also known as B1, thiamin plays a part in a lot of our body functions, including our muscles and nervous system. It's also* *involved with electrolyte flow, enzymatic processes, and the production of hydrochloric acid, which aids in digestion and the metabolism of carbohydrate. A severe deficiency can cause beriberi and can affect the gastrointestinal tract, brain, nervous system, heart, and muscles. Sources include whole-grain cereals, yeast, wheat, beans, lentils, oats, rice, seeds, milk, nuts, pork, and oranges.*

Zinc—*Found in whole grains, fortified cereals, beans, peas, lentils, nut, seeds, tempeh, and tofu, zinc is involved in controlling blood sugar, helps with wound healing and is important to our immune systems.*

B12—*This vitamin is essential to our bodies making red blood cells. It's also important for nerve function. If we have a B12 deficiency, we can suffer from nerve damage and/or anemia. B12 is found in animal products, as well as fortified cereals, hemp and rice milk, meat substitutes, and nutritional yeast.*

But let's not ignore another important question. How easy is it to follow a gluten-free diet? Not very. Eliminating gluten from the diet requires a significant amount of change and a bit of work. Many of us would feel deprived and perhaps even a bit frustrated by the diet. And again, it might also be difficult for some of us to get enough of the nutrition that we all benefit from. Let's take a look at what foods can be included on a gluten-free diet:

Fresh eggs

Majority of dairy products

Natural, unprocessed nuts, seeds, and beans

Fresh poultry, fish, and meats—not breaded, marinated, or battered

Vegetables and fruit

In addition to the above, I like the Mayo Clinic's comprehensive list of grains that can also be a part of this diet:

Amaranth

Arrowroot

Buckwheat

Corn and cornmeal

Flax

Gluten-free flours (rice, soy, corn, potato, bean)

Hominy (corn)

Millet

Quinoa

Rice

Sorghum

Soy

Tapioca

Teff

The permitted foods are a decent list. But we've only buttered one side of the bread. Let's flip it over and review the foods that must be eliminated.

In addition to wheat, rye, triticale, and barley, there are many other foods that must be avoided on a gluten-free diet.

And even excluding something as simple as wheat isn't simple at all. There are many names for it. For example, there is more than one type of wheat flour. These include plain, self-rising, enriched, bromated, and phosphate. This can cause some confusion and unwitting consumption. For those of us with true gluten sensitivity or celiac disease, this can bring on very unpleasant results. We could feel side effects by eating only minimal traces of gluten, for example that found in a small crouton.

Foods to Avoid on a Gluten-Free Diet

Barley

Bulgur

Durum flour

Farina

Graham flour

Kamut

Malt, malt flavoring, and malt vinegar

Rye

Semolina

Spelt

Triticale

Not bad, you say? Well, I'm not finished with the list.

There are many items that unless labeled as "gluten-free" or made with gluten-free grains such as rice, soy, or corn, shouldn't be included on a gluten-free diet. Get ready, here's the long list:

Beer

Bread

Candy

Cereal

Crackers and cookies

Croutons

French fries

Gravies

Imitation seafood or meat

Lunch meats (processed)

Matzo

Pasta

Pies and cakes

Poultry (self-basting)

Rice mixes (seasoned)

Salad dressings

Seasoned snack foods like tortilla and potato chips

Soup bases and other soups

Soy sauce and other sauces

Vegetables in sauce

Is your mind reeling? Are you surprised by the amount of foods to exclude? That's certainly understandable. But hold your horses, my friends, because I'm not done yet.

Do you take prescribed or over-the-counter (OTC) medications and vitamins? Guess what? Some vitamins and medications have gluten in them. It's used as a binding agent. And I've already listed malt flavoring as an item to avoid, but there are other food additives that need to be excluded, including modified food starch.

Cross-Contamination Calamity

Have you heard about cross-contamination? That's when unwanted things can get mixed into food products—for example, during growing, processing, or preparation. This can happen a lot. Because of this, oats—unless they're labeled gluten-free—should be off the table for those who need to adhere to this diet.

There are other gluten-free items that can be cross-contaminated with gluten by the manufacturer or by ourselves. So it's essential to read the ingredients list on nutrition facts labels (more on this in later chapters) and clean utensils and other eating and cooking instruments thoroughly. It's also important to maintain separation of gluten and gluten-free products through all processes of food preparation. This type of diligence is important everywhere we eat, including at home, work, school, restaurants, and more.

To Gluten or Not to Gluten, That Is the Question

As you can see, a gluten-free diet can be challenging. So I must ask, unless you have to follow it because of a specific condition, why would you want to go on such a restrictive diet? It's meant to help with a disease, not for weight loss.

There are many gluten-free diet books available. As I write this, you get around 9,178 results on Amazon when searching "gluten-free diet." Narrowing it down to "gluten-free weight loss," you get about 884 books to choose from. Again, weight loss isn't the point here. Check out the books if you need them for health reasons. Some are quite good and provide helpful tips, support and recipes. But not all of them are written by people in the medical community or other experts. I recommend making sound choices on whose advice you take.

Elaine Monarch, founder and former executive director of the Celiac Disease Foundation, explained why in the following letter about Fox host Elisabeth Hasselbeck's book *The G-free Diet: A Gluten-Free Survival Guide.*

Celiac Colleagues:

I am writing to call your attention to the current publicity surrounding the new book, The G-free Diet: A Gluten-Free Survival Guide *by*

Elisabeth Hasselbeck, co-host of The View. *While it is important to call attention to celiac disease, the information must be accurate—the inaccuracies in this book are potentially dangerous and detrimental to celiacs and to those yet to be diagnosed if people self diagnose and start eating GF. Our mission is to assist in getting people accurately diagnosed, and the message in this book could defeat this mission. It appears that this book is being marketed as a fitness diet—eat g-free and feel so much better. Celiac is incorrectly referred to as an allergy, not an autoimmune disease. The GF diet is the medically mediated prescription that controls the condition for a diagnosed celiac. Several items in the book are misleading and inaccurate and place further limitations on the GF diet. The gluten-free lifestyle is a lifelong commitment for the diagnosed celiac, not an option, not a fad diet—adhering to the GF lifestyle requires patience and persistence. This lifestyle cannot be trivialized.*

Thank you.

Elaine Monarch

Celiac Disease Foundation

Founder and Executive Director

Well said. I counsel people with celiac disease and many more with other gastrointestinal conditions. They have issues that must be addressed and specific diets they need to follow.

I also speak with quite a few people every year about weight management. Many have tried or want to try all different types of diets, including gluten-free. Some have gone on variations of it, for example by avoiding just wheat. Let's investigate these further.

Who Are You Calling Wheat Belly?

The wheat-belly diet is thus named because it calls for its followers to eliminate wheat from their diets. Why, you ask? The author, William Davis, MD, contends, "*wheat is so addictive that it causes uncontrollable eating and produces withdrawal symptoms when you stop consuming it.*" He also suggests that giving up wheat may cure type 2 diabetes, asthma, acid reflux, joint pain, and insomnia. Dr. Davis believes wheat and the products containing wheat are largely to blame for the obesity epidemic. I beg to differ.

First of all, at this time there's no cure for type 2 (or type 1) diabetes. It can be managed, but not cured. And whole wheat has positive attributes. It's a good source of fiber, which among other things, can help slow the absorption of sugar into the blood. So it can actually help control blood sugar. And guess what else? Fiber can help keep us full. It can result in us eating less and help with weight loss.

The reality is that losing those extra pounds can help manage certain diseases. Losing 5 to 10 percent of your total body weight can be beneficial even if you need to lose more.

But we don't need to eliminate wheat to accomplish this.

A Harvard-led study found a lower mortality rate among those who included whole grains in their diet. Researchers estimate that early death risk is reduced by 5 percent overall and by 9 percent from heart disease for every one ounce serving of whole grains eaten.

Dr. Davis discusses central obesity (aka visceral adipose tissue). Let's just call it hidden belly fat. This fat isn't visible like our "beer bellies" and "muffin tops." It resides inside our bodies around our internal organs like the abdomen, heart, and the liver. Not ideal.

The potential negative consequences of this type of obesity are very real. Hidden belly fat increases inflammation in our body. It can raise our chances of heart disease, stroke, high blood pressure, high cholesterol, insulin resistance, dementia, and breast cancer. But there's no evidence that wheat is the culprit. In fact, there's no food or food group that's the sole cause. Belly fat comes from eating too many calories and not exercising enough.

Data from the Framingham Cohort Study found that those who ate two servings of refined grains and three servings of whole grains each day had the *lowest* amount of hidden belly fat.

As is true of gluten-free books, there are tons of other reads about just going wheat-free. If you have a real reason to eliminate wheat from your diet, explore this issue more. It may help you. But if this isn't the case, I say move on.

LISA TILLINGER JOHANSEN

FOUR

Protein Power

"For the vast majority of dieters, diets are short-lived, white-knuckled affairs that, regardless of their actually dietary edicts, can be fairly described as planned suffering. And therein lies the rub."

—Yoni Freedhoff, MD, assistant professor of family medicine and founder and medical director of the Bariatric Medical Institute at the University of Ottawa

Are you a carnivore? Do you like all that animal protein has to offer? Does red meat, poultry, fish, and the like make your mouth water? Perhaps you're a bit more discerning like me. Red meat hasn't touched my lips in over thirty-five years, but I enjoy poultry, low-fat and nonfat cheese, egg whites, a whole egg every now and then, tofu, and more. Or maybe you eschew all animal products. We're all unique and will make different choices.

Protein Proliferation

Regardless of our protein preferences, many of us, particularly in the United States, eat too much of it. And I'm not talking about those who are on a high-protein diet. For a lot of us, if we're having five to seven ounces of meat, fish, poultry, or nonmeat protein sources in a meal, instead of in the whole day, we're overconsuming protein. Has your jaw dropped to the floor?

A reasonable amount of protein for most people is about one ounce for breakfast and two to three ounces each for lunch and dinner. This is for both genders. One ounce is equivalent to one whole egg, two egg whites, one string cheese, or a quarter cup of cottage cheese. Three ounces is the size of a small palm, a deck of cards, or a quarter of the plate. Perhaps many of you are thinking surely that's not enough. For most of us it is.

We get protein from a variety of sources, including:

Eggs

Grains

Legumes

Meat, fish, and poultry

Milk, cheese, and yogurt

Nuts, nut butters, and seeds

Some fruits and vegetables

Tofu

So smooth out that furrowed brow. Rest assured, if we eat balanced meals we should get enough protein. A side note here: there are certain conditions that require higher protein intake. For example, a kidney patient undergoing dialysis has increased protein needs. For those of us who've been told we're protein deficient or for other reasons require more protein, I recommend working with your health care team on an individualized menu plan.

Our bodies use protein for a variety of things. It's found in our cells, tissues, and organs. As part of the digestion process, amino acids, the building blocks of protein, are broken down and used to replace our body proteins. What benefit do we get from protein? It helps:

- *Build and replace muscles, blood, and hair.*

- *Keep organs and muscles healthy.*

- *Maintain normal body functions.*

There are 20 amino acids. The body makes some, but not all of them. The amino acids that we don't make are called essential amino acids.

Complete proteins contain all of the essential amino acids. Eggs, meat, poultry, fish, milk, and cheese fall in

this category.

Incomplete proteins are low in one or more of the amino acids. But there's a way to improve this by adding in a complementary protein. The two together, like rice and beans, form a complete protein. But, contrary to popular belief, we don't have to eat the complementary proteins in the same meal. Just eat them in the same day.

The Perils of Protein

Why is it important that we not get too much protein? Does it really matter? It sure can.

Animal protein can be tough on the kidneys. It also stresses the liver. These hardworking organs do a lot of things for us, including handling the excess nitrogen we get from our protein intake.

Too much protein can be damaging for those who have kidney disease (not on dialysis) or who are at risk of decreased kidney function. I work with a lot of renal patients and I make sure that they aren't overconsuming it. If you're saying to yourself this doesn't apply to you because your kidneys are fine, think again.

In the United States, around twenty million people are at risk for kidney function decline, *but don't know it*. And in the early stages of kidney disease, there often aren't any symptoms. I see many people who aren't aware they have a problem until they're in stage three, which is moderate decline. There are five stages of kidney disease. Once you reach stage five, you're looking at dialysis or transplant.

People at increased risk of kidney damage include those with high blood pressure or diabetes, or who are sixty-five or older. Not you, you say? I just told you how many people are at risk for decreased kidney function. Now let's talk about diabetes.

Sugar Shock

Approximately 347 million people have diabetes worldwide. India has the most cases—about forty million. This number is projected to increase to sixty-nine million by 2025. There are many other countries with a high rate of this disease. And as can happen with a variety of conditions, we're not always aware we have an issue. For example, of the close to twenty-six million Americans with diabetes, seven million don't even know they have it.

Our blood sugar can also be above the normal range (70 to 99 fasting, less than 140 two hours after eating), but not yet at the diabetic level. This is termed prediabetes. About seventy-nine million people twenty and older in the United States are prediabetic. Many likely don't know that their blood glucose levels are higher than normal. I call prediabetes "diet controlled diabetes." The majority of prediabetics graduate to diabetes.

Protein, We Have a Problem

We can also put ourselves at risk for osteoporosis when we eat too much animal protein. It causes us to excrete more calcium via the kidneys than normal, which can be harmful to our bones. Countries that have lower-protein diets have decreased incidence of osteoporosis and hip fractures.

Increased calcium excretion has a ripple effect. It raises our risk for kidney stones. In addition, researchers in the United Kingdom found that adding five additional ounces of fish to a "normal diet" increased the risk of getting urinary tract stones by as much as 250 percent.

Too much protein in the diet can also put us at a higher risk for colon cancer, as well as other cancers. High-protein diets can also cause ketones. These occur when the body has to break down fat for energy or fuel, which often happens with high-protein, low-carbohydrate diets. Carbohydrate is our body's main energy source, and when we don't get enough we can go into a state of ketosis (having ketones). This can make our kidneys have to work too hard. It can also cause us to lose water, which accounts for a lot of the initial weight loss.

Extra water is required to metabolize the excessive protein eaten. The quick weight shed that occurs is water loss, not fat, as you become dehydrated. This is the premise of many diets, including the one-day diet, which promises weight loss of two to five pounds in one day. Come again?

Do you really think that we can lose that many real pounds in one day? If you do, I'd like to sell you a bridge...Since its followers drink protein water all day long, it's no wonder that weight loss occurs. But once you rehydrate, the lost pounds suddenly return.

Another diet that relies on ketosis is the Lindora diet. Founded in 1971 by Dr. Marshall Stamper, Lindora can be accessed online and through walk-in clinics. It's a low-calorie, low-carb, high-protein diet that advertises its followers will lose 10 percent of their total body weight in ten weeks. On their website's "You have questions—We have answers" section, they say that ketosis is "misunderstood." That's what they want you to think. Don't fall for it.

Studies have also shown that we can experience problems when our bodies have to break down the essential amino acid methionine. Methionine turns into the sulfur-containing amino acid homocysteine in the body. Homocysteine can put us at increased risk for heart disease, stroke, blood clots, depression, dementia, and Alzheimer's.

Our bodies like to be in balance. I equate it to a seesaw. There's a person sitting on either end in perfect alignment. That's how we want to be, nice and even. When we do something like put ourselves in a state of ketosis, someone gets off the seesaw and we tilt. We're out of whack.

I pepper my classes and consults with visuals. One of them is telling my clients that the human body's like a big lake dotted with our internal parts and surrounded by our external ones. We're squishy. In fact, the adult body is about 60 percent water and likes it that way. When we lose too much water, we run the risk of dehydration, which can also put pressure on the kidneys and the heart.

What's Up, What's Down?

There are many diet books available on the low-carb, high-protein diet. Atkins, Sugar Busters, the Zone, Protein Power, and the Dukan diet are some on a very lengthy list. Some, like the Body-*for*-LIFE diet, aren't low-carbohydrate, but are still high-protein. The Paleo Diet is a high-protein diet, but it also embraces an increased level of exclusion. It warrants its own section in this chapter.

The basics of the high-protein, low-carbohydrate diet are, well, more protein, less carb. Certain foods are off the table. Less-healthy choices of acceptable foods often aren't. Some have other restrictions, such as Body-*for*-LIFE, which calls for daily weigh-ins and a meal that must be eaten within sixty minutes' time. Most claim that their diet will result in quick weight loss—a sure sign of a fad diet.

Dietary breakdown recommendations by the Institute of Medicine are 20–35 percent of calories from protein, 45–65 percent from carbohydrate and 10–35 percent from fat. Barring specific dietary needs, I usually recommend 15 to 20 percent protein, 45 to 50 percent carbohydrate and 30 percent fat.

The various diets have different protein and carbohydrate ratios. Depending on the author, there are also divergent takes on which foods are acceptable and which aren't. Typically, these types of diets can be poor, nutritionally speaking. They can be low in certain vitamins (like A and C), fiber, and calcium. And while many of them suggest taking vitamins to make up for any deficiencies, it's best for us to try and get our vitamins and minerals through food. That's what our bodies like best.

Approximately 40 percent of Americans take multivitamins, at a whopping annual cost of about $28 billion. Several 2013 studies pointed to the lack of effectiveness in taking them. Among the findings, it was reported that multivitamins didn't lead to preventing heart disease, cancer, early death, or cognitive decline.

Steven Salzberg, MD, a professor of medicine at Johns Hopkins, said of the results: "I think this is a great example of how our intuition leads us astray. It seems reasonable that if a little bit of something is good for you, then more should be better for you. It's not true. Supplementation with extra vitamins or micronutrients doesn't really benefit you if you don't have a deficiency."

Your doctor can determine if you have a vitamin or mineral deficiency and prescribe a course of treatment.

If you want to take a multivitamin, I don't recommend taking one with more than 100 percent of the recommended daily allowance (RDA). And tell your health care provider about all the OTC medications you're taking. He or she can make sure you're not taking something that you shouldn't because it might not mix well with your other medications or a condition that you have.

Another area to review with regard to a high-protein diet, or any diet for that matter is exercise. Our bodies like and need it. Some of the high-protein and low-carbohydrate diets, like Atkins, don't include it as a recommendation, but do acknowledge its importance in weight maintenance. Others suggest varying types and amounts of exercise, from the Dukan diet's twenty minutes per day to Body-*for*-LIFE's forty-five minutes of weight training three times per week (alternating with twenty minutes of aerobic exercise three days per week). The Protein Power diet prefers more weight-resistance exercises to aerobic activity.

The 2010 Dietary Guidelines for Americans, issued by the Department of Agriculture and the Department of Health and Human Services, recommends thirty minutes of aerobic physical activity most days of the week for adults and sixty minutes for children and adolescents. For adults wanting to lose weight, go for sixty minutes most days of the week. Resistance training is recommended twice a week for fifteen to twenty minutes. The 2015 Dietary Guidelines Advisory Committee maintained this recommendation.

Many of the authors of the high-protein, low-carb diets make health claims. They say that in addition to weight loss, their diet plans can also help combat high blood pressure, heart disease, diabetes, and more. Weight loss, when needed, can certainly help manage chronic diseases and other important things. I've already touched on this. But as discussed earlier in this chapter, too much or too little of a food group may not be good for us. For example, a diabetic on medication to lower blood sugar who severely restricts carbohydrates could experience low blood sugar episodes (hypoglycemia). This can be extremely serious and may even be life threatening.

The myriad of high-protein, low-carb diets out there have similarities and differences. Let's take a look at some of the mechanics:

Diet	Protein	Carbo-hydrate	Fat	Exclusions	Vitamin Y/N
Atkins	All choices okay. 3 servings of 4 to 6 ounces daily.	Uses "net carbs" concept in which fiber grams are sub-tracted from grams of total carb. **Phase 1:** 20 grams of net carbs per day (primarily from veggies	All fat, even satur-ated fat is fine.	**Induction Phase:** Most fruit, bread, pasta, grains, high-sugar baked goods, nuts, and alcohol.	Y
Beach Body 21 Day Fix	30 percent of total daily calories.	40 percent of total daily calories.	30 percent of total daily calories.	Almond, soy, and coconut milk, coconut water and fruit juice 3 times a week only in exchange for one yellow container.	Y

Diet	Protein	Carbo-hydrate	Fat	Exclusions	Vitamin Y/N
Body-_for-_ LIFE	45 percent to 50 percent of total daily calories.	45 to 50 percent of total daily calories.	1–2 tbsp of healthy oil,	Bacon, hot dogs, fatty cuts of meat, fried meat, lard, butter, mayo, coconut oil, whole dairy, concentrate sweets, chips, white rice, soda.	Y
Carbo-hydrate Addicts	**2 Comple-mentary Meals include:** 3–4 ounces most meats, poultry, or fish; 2 eggs or 2 ounces of cheese or 1/2 cup cottage cheese.	**2 Comple-mentary Meals include:** 2 cups of allowed vege-tables. Milk as indi-cated in protein column.	**2 Comple-mentary Meals include:** 1–2 tbsp of fat.	Broccoli, brussels sprouts, carrots, legumes, and only small amounts of onion. No snacking in between meals.	Y

85

Diet	Protein	Carbo-hydrate	Fat	Exclusions	Vitamin Y/N
Carbo-hydrate Addicts	Up to 2 ounces of milk daily. **1 Reward Meal:** Can have anything, but must be eaten within 60 minutes' time.	**1 Reward Meal:** Can have anything, but must be eaten within 60 minutes' time.	**1 Reward Meal:** Can have anything, but must be eaten within 60 minutes' time.		

Diet	Protein	Carbo-hydrate	Fat	Exclusions	Vitamin Y/N
Dukan	Over 40 percent of total daily calories. **All Stages:** Unlimited protein (no pork or lamb in first two stages). **Cruise Stage:** Add 1 serving of hard cheese. **Stabili-zation Stage:**	**All Stages:** 1.5 tbsp of oat bran. **Attack Stage:** Approxi-mately 27 percent of total calories. Only 4 grams of daily fiber. **Cruise Stage:** Approxi-mately 38 percent of total calories. Unlimited servings of 28 non-starchy veggies.	20 percent from total daily calories.	**Attack Stage:** Everything but protein, oat bran, and water. **Cruise Stage:** Corn, carrots, peas, and potatoes.	Y

Diet	Protein	Carbo-hydrate	Fat	Exclusions	Vitamin Y/N
Dukan	Eat what you like, but follow all-protein plan in **Attack Stage** 1 day per week.	2 tbsp of oat bran. Only 11 grams of daily fiber. **Consoli-dation Stage:** 2 slices of whole-grain bread, 1 piece of fruit, 1–2 servings of starch. 1–2 "cele-bration" meals, in which you can eat whatever you want, are included per week.			

Diet	Protein	Carbo-hydrate	Fat	Exclusions	Vitamin Y/N
Dukan		**Stabili-zation Stage:** 3 tbsp of oat-bran daily. Eat what you like, but one day per week follow the Phase 1 meal plan.			
Protein Power	Calcu-lated per individual.	Weight Loss: 20 to 40 grams a day.	No limit.	Excludes grains. Limits/elimi-nates starchy veggies, legumes,	Y

Diet	Protein	Carbo-hydrate	Fat	Exclusions	Vitamin Y/N
Protein Power		Tran-sition: 50 grams per day. Main-tenance: 70 to 130 grams a day. 25 grams of fiber per day.		concen-trated sweets, certain fruits like mangos and pineapple.	
Scars-dale	43 percent of total daily calories	34.5 percent of total daily calories	22.5 percent of total daily calories	3 meals per day only. No snacks. No milk or starchy vegetables. Strict menu. Very low-calorie diet.	

Diet	Protein	Carbo-hydrate	Fat	Exclusions	Vitamin Y/N
South Beach	Encourages eating lean protein. Around 20 percent of total daily calories.	Depending on the phase, about 28 percent to 40 percent of total daily calories. Doesn't count carbs, but encourages low sugar and low glycemic index choices.	About 40 percent of total daily calories. Encourages healthy fats.	First 2 weeks: Fruit, bread, cereal, corn, rice, and pasta. Moving forward, rice, potatoes, beets, and corn continue to be strongly discouraged. No alcohol. No sugary desserts. In later phases, alcohol can be introduced, but is limited. Bans unhealthy fats.	Y

Diet	Protein	Carbo-hydrate	Fat	Exclusions	Vitamin Y/N
Sugar Busters	Approximately 30 percent of total daily calories. Recommends dividing body weight by 2.2 to get daily protein grams.	40 percent of total daily calories.	30 percent of total daily calories. Emphasis on mono- and polyunsaturated fats.	Refined flours, sugar, baked beans, corn, potatoes, beets, carrots, raisins, ripe bananas, white rice, pasta, bread, bacon, fried chicken, most cold cuts, molasses, corn syrup, sugary sodas, honey, and beer. Not for avid exercisers.	Y
Zone	30 percent of total daily calories.	40 percent of total daily calories.	30 percent of total daily calories.		Y

Diet	Protein	Carbo-hydrate	Fat	Exclusions	Vitamin Y/N
Zone	Protein at every meal and snack.	"Favor-able" carbs include most fruits and vege-tables, as well as lentils, beans, and whole grains.		Small Amounts of "Unfavor-able" carbs: bread, bagels, dry cereal, tortillas, brown rice, pasta, papaya, mango, banana, carrots, fruit juices. Low-fat and nonfat cheese and milk preferred over whole fat versions. Egg whites and egg substitutes preferred over whole eggs.	

For royal watchers, it's been reported that Kate Middleton followed the Dukan diet, the popular French weight-loss plan described above, to lose pounds before her nuptials to Prince William. As a result, it's also been called the "princess diet."

One of the best-selling diet books of all time, *The Complete Scarsdale Medical Diet*, was made a bit infamous by the murder of its creator, cardiologist Herman Tarnower, MD. His long-term girlfriend shot him in his home with his own gun in 1980. It wasn't because of the restrictive nature of his proposed diet. Apparently she didn't like his philandering ways. And while not grounds for murder, the Scarsdale diet is murderous. Recently, the Healthy Weight Forum highlighted a typical day's diet on this plan:

Breakfast

- *Slice of whole meal or protein toast (no butter or spreads)*
- *A half grapefruit. If not available, then half of a mango, papaya, or cantaloupe, 1 cup diced fresh pineapple or a big slice of casaba, honeydew, or other melon*
- *Coffee (no milk or sugar)*

Lunch

- *Canned tuna*
- *Salad (example: lettuce, tomato, celery, and cucumbers) with oil-free dressing*
- *Water, coffee, tea, or diet soda*

Dinner

- *Roast chicken, turkey, lamb (all visible fat removed), fish, shellfish, or vegetable protein*
- *Salad with vinegar and lemon dressing*
- *Coffee*

Beverages

- *Water (at least four glasses per day), soda water, diet drinks, tea*

Not only is this restrictive diet boring, it can put us at risk for certain diseases. Even as far back as its inception in the 1970s, Dr. Tarnower recommended that the dieter only follow it for about two weeks, then switch to his more liberal Keep Trim program. Tarnower also recommended walking every day.

As discussed, when we embark upon a high-protein, low-carbohydrate diet, we can put ourselves in a state of ketosis. It may sound good to break down your stored body fat to use as energy, but it's like robbing Peter to pay Paul. Something eventually gives. And guess what, along with the water weight loss, which translates to happiness when you weigh yourself, you also can lose muscle. Some people also suffer from constipation, fatigue, headaches, insomnia, dry mouth, and bad breath due to ketosis. Is it good to have such unwanted side effects from our daily diet? I say no.

The term "ketogenic diet" can be used to describe any low-carb diet that causes ketosis on a regular basis. The original ketogenic diet was used to manage epilepsy in children. The medical version of this diet is a high-fat one at a ratio of four to one in fat to carbohydrate and protein. Side effects can include irregular periods, kidney stones, and high amounts of calcium in the urine. No one should go on a ketogenic diet without first consulting with their doctor.

Authors of popular diets make some interesting statements in interviews and in their own writings. Here's my response to some of the late Dr. Atkins's remarks:

Atkins: *Well, I would never do a study because I'm a practicing physician. I mean, all I do is treat people.*

Johansen: *It's definitely important to treat people. We all need medical attention at some point or another. But we also benefit from scientific studies for so many aspects of health care, including gaining a better understanding of cause-and-effect relationships with regard to diet. And they can help us live longer and healthier.*

Atkins: *You take the healthiest diet in the world, if you gave those people vitamins, they would be twice as healthy. So vitamins are valuable.*

Johansen: *We typically can get the vitamins we need from our food. That's why it's important to eat balanced meals. If we need to take a* *vitamin to make up for the inadequacies of our limited diets, then we're not doing something right.*

Atkins: *I think I can wipe out diabetes.*

Johansen: *So how'd that go?*

Studies have shown that high-protein, low-carbohydrate diets don't result in greater weight loss than a typical higher carbohydrate diet. Most participants gain back the weight they lose no matter which diet they're on. Other studies have shown that those on Atkins for two years lost on average almost nine pounds. We can also do this, and more, on a healthier eating plan.

Several major studies have highlighted the negative health impacts of high-protein, low-carb diets. This includes data compiled for many years from over thirty-seven thousand males in the Health Professionals Follow-Up Study and over eighty-three thousand females from the Nurses' Health Study that found eating both unprocessed and processed red meat resulted in increased cases of type 2 diabetes, cancer and cardiovascular disease, as well as a higher risk of premature death.

Our kidneys and colons aren't the only organs that can be affected by consuming too much protein. Let's take a look at our hearts. If we're choosing less healthy proteins like red meat or eating the skin on poultry, we're ingesting a lot of saturated fat and calories. This isn't good for us.

The 2015 *Dietary Guidelines Advisory Committee* suggested dialing back the decades-long recommendation to limit daily cholesterol intake from food to 300 mg (200 mg with heart disease). This is because studies have shown that cholesterol from food may only slightly impact our blood cholesterol, which can affect our heart health. But remember one size doesn't fit all. We're all different and some of us have diseases or genetic predispositions that would still have us benefit from a low-cholesterol diet. I recommend you speak with your health care provider for guidance.

Regardless, it's best to be moderate. And take note, saturated fat is still something that we need to limit. It's not heart healthy.

Researchers at Greece's University of Athens Medical School looked at the diets of forty-three thousand women in Sweden age thirty to forty-nine over a sixteen-year period. They found that those who followed a high-protein, low-carbohydrate diet had a 5 percent increased risk of developing heart disease. At the conclusion of the study, 1,270 of the women in the study group had been diagnosed with cardiovascular disease. And a study published in the *New England Journal of Medicine* concluded that a diet high in unrefined carbohydrate and low in fat resulted in the lowest number of blockages in the coronary arteries, while high-protein, low-carbohydrate diets resulted in the most.

Fat, Fat, and More Fat

In Sweden, Annika Dahlqvist, MD, was investigated for violations after suggesting a high-fat, low-carb diet to her patients. She was cleared. Still, I don't recommend her diet, which calls for its followers to eat full-fat dairy products and leave the fat on meats. Its stoplight color approach has green, amber, and red-light foods. These are:

Green-Light Foods
(freely allowed)

Meat, fish, eggs
Vegetables
Natural yogurt, cheese, cream, and butter
Olive oil and canola oil
Homemade sauces

Amber-Light Foods
(moderate consumption)

Fruit (except for dried fruit)
Nuts and seeds
Lentils and beans
Chocolate with 65 percent to 95 percent quantity of cocoa

Red-Light Foods
(limited consumption)

Sugary drinks
Dried fruit
Desserts
Products containing rice, bread, flour, potato, and corn
Cereal, biscuits, pasta, pastry, and like starches
Margarine
Sunflower, safflower, soybean, peanut, corn, and other omega-6 based oils

High-fat items, particularly with saturated fat, aren't heart healthy. I always tell my clients that no one over age two should drink whole milk or eat foods that have it as an ingredient. (A possible exception would be if they're underweight). And encouraging people not to trim off visible fat from meats is concerning. While I agree with limiting or avoiding sugary drinks, desserts, and margarine (unless trans-fat free), I don't agree with avoiding quality starches, particularly whole grains.

Are We Cavemen?

The Paleo Diet suggests that we should eat more like our ancestors. I don't mean our great-grandparents or even our great-great ones. We need to go back a lot further, over ten thousand years ago, before the agricultural revolution. That's very far down on the family tree. We're talking about hunter-gatherers. Foods on this diet include fish, meat, poultry, eggs, nuts, fruits, and vegetables. It doesn't allow grains, sugar, dairy, legumes, potatoes, processed oils, or more modern foods (ten thousand years or younger). The reasoning is that our bodies are genetically mapped to eat like they did so many years ago.

This diet consists of about 38 percent of calories from protein, 23 percent from carbohydrate and 39 percent from fat. This is considered to be a high-protein, high-fat, low-carb diet.

There are different versions of the diet. Some are a bit more flexible and allow processed oils from nuts and fruits. Others restrict nightshade vegetables like eggplant and tomato or recommend eating raw foods and fasting. But the basic tenets remain.

Let's look at the bottom of fitness author Mark Sisson's pyramid from his book *The Primal Blueprint*. It isn't grains like we're used to seeing. His consists of meat, fish, fowl, and eggs called the "bulk of dietary calories." The next level of the pyramid is organic or locally grown vegetables. Among the moderate foods to eat near the top of the pyramid is high-fat, raw, fermented, and unpasteurized milk. Sisson calls his tenets "laws."

For the record, pasteurization kills bacteria that can cause illnesses such as diphtheria, tuberculosis, listeriosis, and typhoid fever. It actually can save lives. Raw or unpasteurized milk doesn't provide the same protection.

And when we limit dairy and grains, we lose out on the nutrients they offer. Calcium, fiber, phosphorus, and vitamin D are just a few. Our intestinal health, bowel regularity, bones, muscle function, and protection from certain diseases such as cancer and heart disease could take a hit. And again, for those with certain conditions—like someone who has kidney disease and isn't on dialysis—it's too much protein. Someone with diabetes who's on medications to lower blood sugar wouldn't get enough carbohydrates, which can result in hypoglycemia. Remember, carbohydrates are our most efficient energy source.

In addition, the Paleo Diet includes a lot of fat. And depending on the type of protein eaten, much of it could be of the saturated type. This isn't heart healthy.

To combat some of its nutritional deficiencies, part of the Paleo Diet suggests taking a vitamin D supplement if you're not getting midday sunshine without sunscreen at least thirty minutes several times a week. Calcium is also sometimes recommended, as is fish oil if you don't eat a lot of fish or shellfish. A diet that may require supplements to ensure we get enough of necessary vitamins and minerals isn't a good one.

While cavemen didn't have a lot of the lifestyle diseases that we have today, they didn't live as long as we do either. The average Paleolithic era person lived to the ripe old age of eighteen. And cardiovascular disease did exist. But they had better teeth than our more modern species. There's a lesson. Let's improve our dental hygiene.

People do lose weight on the Paleo Diet. It was recently reported that John M. Brown, a six-foot-one male, lost 130 pounds on the Paleo Diet. He went from 370 pounds to 240 pounds. He's not done yet. His goal is to reach 220 pounds.

In March 2015, British singer and Grammy winner Sam Smith posted a picture on Instagram letting everyone know he lost fourteen pounds in fourteen days. That's an astonishing and unhealthy pound a day. He credits Amelia Freer, nutritional therapist and author of *Eat. Nourish. Glow.* for his weight loss. Freer describes her diet as "gluten, dairy, and refined-sugar free," and says it's "most closely aligned with the paleo concept."

And 2016 US presidential hopeful and former Florida governor Jeb Bush recently let the world know he joined the paleo craze. He explained this was the reason he no longer put barbecue sauce on his meat. Those reporting the story seemed more concerned on how Bush would manage this diet while campaigning across the country. It appears that he did face a few obstacles on the road. At one point, Bush chowed down on pie at a political meeting.

My husband definitely lives partly, culinarily speaking only, in the Paleolithic Age. His brown diet? It's mostly meat. He chooses very few fruits and veggies. He doesn't typically include healthy grains, opting for less nutritious carbohydrate fare. He's not a very healthy eater and should improve his diet. Luckily for him, due to good genes his health hasn't suffered for it...yet.

But ever the good wife, I'm looking out for him. He eats more fruits and veggies than he thinks he does. I hide them in stews, casseroles, and more.

Where's That Beef?

There are diets out there that take the opposite approach of the high-protein, low-carbohydrate diet. *The Starch Solution* proposes a diet that consists of 70 percent starch, 0 percent meat and dairy, 10 percent fruit and 20 percent veggies. This is a vegan diet. No animal products allowed.

According to John A. MacDougall, MD, one of the authors, "Basic to our human nature is the scientific fact that we're, and have always been, primarily starch eaters." He adds that over the past thirteen thousand years and beyond, starch has been the main focus of all "healthy, large, successful populations." He cites China, Japan, most other Asian countries, Aztecs, Mayans, Incans, and ancient Egyptians, as well as the Europeans. He backs this up with the fact that starch grains have been found in grinding tools that date back to the Paleolithic period in the Czech Republic, Russia, and Italy. MacDougall also points out that the chimpanzee, a close relative of humans, is pretty much a vegetarian.

Dean Ornish, MD, is also a proponent of the vegetarian lifestyle. His reversal diet excludes most animal products except for yogurt, nonfat milk, and egg whites. It consists of 70 percent to 75 percent carbohydrate, 10 percent fat (primarily monounsaturated and polyunsaturated), 15 percent to 20 percent protein and 5 mg of cholesterol daily. It's loaded with fruits and veggies.

It's called the reversal diet because it has been shown to reverse heart disease. Dr. Ornish's Lifestyle Heart Trial found that people who followed the reversal diet had fewer blockages in their coronary arteries. Many studies find that vegetarians have lower risk of obesity, hypertension, diabetes, heart disease, lung, colon and breast cancers, gallstones, and diverticular disease. Skipping animal products may also be associated with a reduced risk of osteoporosis and better kidney function.

It's rare that I'm able to get anyone interested in discussing a vegetarian diet. More often than not, they say it's too restrictive. The majority of people don't want to cut out meat. But if you want to try it out, there's a range of vegetarianism. Maybe one of these would be palatable to you:

Vegan—*Eats no dairy, eggs, red meat, seafood, poultry, pork, or animal byproducts.*

Lacto-Ovo—*Eats no red meat, seafood, poultry, or pork, but will have eggs and dairy.*

Lacto—*Restricts animal products, but will have dairy.*

Ovo—*Restricts animal product, but will have eggs.*

Pesco/Pesca—*Doesn't eat red meat, poultry or pork, but will have fish.*

Pollo—*Eats poultry, but no red meat, pork, or seafood.*

Semi or Flexitarian—*Will from time to time eat red meat, seafood, poultry, or pork.*

Fruitarian—*Eats raw fruit, nuts, and grains.*

I haven't eaten red meat or pork for many years, but will

have poultry and seafood. I'm a version of the semi or flexitarian vegetarian.

My clients show much more interest in the Mediterranean diet, a heart healthy way to eat. The Lyon Diet Heart Study found that followers of this plan were less likely to have a heart attack. Further, they had a decreased risk of dying an early death from any cause. The diet includes animal protein, but limits meat, particularly beef, lamb, and pork, to one to two times per month. Calories from fat are reasonable—olive oil and canola oil are the suggested sources. It includes moderate amounts of ocean-caught fish, recommending at least two servings per week. It focuses on fruits, vegetables, whole grains, peas, beans, lentils, nuts, seeds, and tofu. Five or more servings of veggies and two to four servings of fruit are recommended daily. Processed foods are discouraged. It's a healthy way to eat.

Another diet that some of my clients embrace is the DASH (Dietary Approaches to Stop Hypertension) diet. Designed to help people lower their blood pressure, it can also be beneficial in managing other conditions. And while not designed for this, it can help us to lose weight. *US News and World Report* named the DASH diet the best for 2014.

This eating plan for life is low in cholesterol, total fat, and saturated fat. It reduces sodium intake and includes four to five daily servings of fruits and vegetables. That's certainly an increase for some of us. It calls for two to three servings of low-fat dairy, six to eight servings of whole grains, six or less servings of fish, poultry, and lean meat, and two to three servings of fat a day. You can have four to five servings of nuts, seeds and legumes a week. It also recommends no more than five servings of sweets per week. So the DASH diet includes lots of fruits and veggies and other healthier food choices and limits fats, sodium, alcohol, added sugar, and excess protein.

Too much protein can put us at risk for a variety of healthy problems. And numerous studies have shown that eating less or no meat can result in better health. One such study, the China-Cornell-Oxford Project, aka the China Project, is considered to be a comprehensive look at the association between diet and disease. It also found harmful health effects from high-protein diets. Because diets among the Chinese people vary from totally plant-based to those containing a lot of animal products, researchers were able to follow this diverse study group for long periods of time and draw important conclusions.

The China Project found that the populations with increased animal products in their diets, even in small amounts, experienced the same type of cancers found in Western populations. Even lean proteins were correlated with increased cancer rates. The closer the diets came to including no animal products, the more the incidence of cancer fell. These nearly vegetarian populations were practically free of not only cancer, but heart attacks as well. Another study that followed thirty-two thousand adults over a six-year period found that even those who ate white meat, but not red meat, had a 300 percent increased rate of colon cancer. This gives me pause, because while I haven't eaten red meat in over thirty-eight years, I do eat poultry. Cancer, including of the colon, runs in my family. So does heart disease. As I write this I'm considering moving toward a more comprehensive vegetarian lifestyle. Dean Ornish, here I come!

There's no clear consensus on white meat vs. dark meat, but fish and poultry are typically considered white meat. Most often, beef, lamb and pork are classified as red meat.

So let me ask you. Does the high-protein, low-carbohydrate diet still sound good to you? It's definitely something to think about. But not in a good way.

FIVE

Running on Empty

"Will substituting lemon juice and pepper for meals lead not to a 'purified' body, but rather one that in the future is so frail, it must reside in a wheelchair?"

—Judith J. Wurtman, PhD, coauthor of *The Serotonin Diet*

Losing weight is a mathematical equation. It's pretty simple: if you put in more calories than you burn, you gain weight. Conversely, if you put in fewer calories than you burn, you lose pounds. Finally, if you put in the same amount of calories that you burn, the scale doesn't budge either way. You maintain your weight. That's all there is to it.

One pound equals 3,500 calories. Cutting 500 calories per day through diet and exercise should result in a one-pound weight loss in a week. If you cut 1,000 calories per day, you should lose two pounds in seven days.

I speak to so many people who want very quick weight loss. While I can certainly understand the desire for fast results, it shouldn't come at the expense of our health. Losing weight too quickly isn't good for us. To do so typically requires greatly cutting back on calories. This usually means we aren't getting enough to keep our bodies running efficiently. But that doesn't stop some from still trying. What's their strategy? Often it's a low-calorie (LCD) or very-low-calorie (VLCD) diet.

There are differing opinions among health care professionals about the role of the LCD and even the VLCD eating plans. If medically monitored and reasonably balanced, some are okay with them. I don't typically embrace them and encourage my clients not to go below 1,200 calories without medical supervision and nutrition education. I like to see people make healthy food choices as part of a weight-loss plan they can carry through for lifelong eating. And of course not all LCDs and VLCDs are alike.

The LCD contains fewer calories than it would take to maintain weight for most adults. It's typically defined as between 1,000 and 1,200 calories. But a daily calorie level greater than 800 or less than 1,200 is considered a LCD.

The VLCD has 800 or fewer daily calories. A moderate to severely obese person could lose three to five pounds per week on this diet. Side effects associated with VLCDs include nausea, diarrhea, fatigue, and constipation. A more serious complication could be gallstones, which can form when we lose weight too quickly—particularly among obese females.

Our bodies have a very important need: energy. I often compare us to cars. What happens to our vehicles if we don't put in enough gasoline? They stop moving. While our bodies don't immediately stop working if we don't put enough calories in our mouths, they don't function as well. And it can put us at risk for nutritional deficiencies, malnutrition, and other things. Keeping the car analogy, how would you like to try going on a long trip with only a quarter tank of gas and nowhere along the way to fill her up? That's our bodies on restricted calories.

Our basal metabolic rate (BMR) is the number of calories our bodies need just to function every day. As

you're reading this book, the very busy factory that is you is working away. The blood is coursing through your veins, arteries, and capillaries. Your heart is beating, your lungs are inflating and deflating, your gastrointestinal system is churning away, your liver is performing functions such as detoxification, your gallbladder is breaking down bile, your kidneys are monitoring your water levels and affecting blood pressure, among other things. Hormones and enzymes are working their magic. And your brain is thinking, your bones are breaking themselves down and rebuilding them, and electrical synapses are communicating things throughout your body. The appendix...well, it's doing nothing, but that's another story.

How much of this do you feel? Not too much. But it's happening and it requires energy to do so. If we don't put enough calories in, our body factory loses efficiency. Something goes on strike.

Replacement Parts

One type of LCD is meal replacement. Most of us know what that is. Typically, several meals are replaced with a shake or a bar and then you have one sensible meal. Perhaps the oldest program is Slim Fast. It's been around since 1977.

Tommy Lasorda, Kathie Lee Gifford, Whoopie Goldberg, Ann Jillian, Shari Belafonte, and Rachel Hunter have all served as its spokespeople.

While it's declined in popularity over the years, with sales revenue dropping by 40 percent since 2008, Slim Fast was still recently ranked number four on *US News & World Report's* Best Commercial Diet list. Weight Watchers, Jenny Craig, and the Biggest Loser beat it out in that order.

There are other meal-replacement diets, including the cookie diet, in which you eat a cookie every couple of hours and then a five-hundred- to seven-hundred-calorie dinner. On this plan, a multivitamin is recommended. Talk about a cookie monster. Special K is also in on the meal-replacement act. You eat two meals with their products and then one sensible meal with items of your choosing.

Another popular plan is Medifast. This is a high-protein, low-carb diet of about 800 to 1,000 calories per day. Low glycemic, kosher, vegetarian, diabetic, and lactose-free plans, among others, are offered. Medifast has seventy products, including shakes, bars, soups, puddings, oatmeal, and chili. The plan has its followers eat five meal replacements and one sensible meal each day. The recommended "lean and green" meal should have lean fish or meat that's either baked, grilled, boiled, poached or broiled, along with a salad or other green vegetables. Of the green veggies, brussels sprouts and peas aren't allowed. I don't know if I could live without brussels sprouts. They're my favorite veggie.

Medifast does encourage exercising regularly and takes into account medical conditions. But besides being very low calorie, it excludes most carbohydrates, which I don't recommend. As with all fad diets, graduating to healthy eating and maintaining the weight loss can be challenging.

Britain has its own version of a popular meal-replacement plan. It's the Tony Ferguson diet. Similar in theory to its American counterparts, it also includes 24/7 access to a hotline for a joining fee.

For many, the structure and convenience of this type of diet is appealing. It doesn't require a lot of planning or thought, making it easy for those who get overwhelmed if there's too much variety. There's often online support available, which is helpful.

But meal-replacement programs also have cons. For one thing, not having enough balanced meals per day containing whole foods can cause us to miss out on important nutrients. In addition, some participants of meal-replacement diets don't find them to be satisfying. They may not feel full after meals.

Another con of these types of programs is that the lack of variety that makes it easy can also make it boring. Studies have shown that long-term success isn't often achieved. This can be exacerbated if there's no nutrition education to provide the skills necessary for putting together healthy, balanced meals.

Sometimes people on these diets may experience side effects. Some who've been on Slim Fast have reported experiencing lightheadedness. And let's also not forget that the products can be costly.

There are certainly cases in which participants are successful in this particular type of diet. An Australian study in the *Journal of Nutrition* found that meal replacements, in this case shakes, were as effective for weight-loss as more "conventional, structured" diet plans. And as it turns out, the study group on the meal replacements had a more positive outlook about dieting and found it to be more convenient than those on the "regular food" plan. But it's likely these individuals won't stay on meal replacements for life and at some point will resume eating regular meals throughout the day. Therefore, it's essential they be taught good eating habits for life so that they successfully navigate this transition.

Courting the Cleanse

Dating back fifty years, the Master Cleanse (aka the lemonade diet and the maple syrup diet) has been a go-to for those looking for quick weight loss. Stanley Burroughs developed it with the idea of detoxifying the body by fasting. Singer Beyoncé gave it some recent headlines when she told the world she'd lost twenty pounds by cleansing.

It's unclear to me why we need to detox with a special elixir. Our amazing bodies have organs that already do this for us: the liver and the kidneys.

This unhealthy diet plan doesn't include any food. Not one bite. All you have is one liquid concoction. The ingredients for one glass are:

10 ounces filtered water
2 tablespoons fresh-squeezed lemon juice
2 tablespoons grade-B organic maple syrup
1/10 teaspoon cayenne pepper

I don't know about you, but I'd be one grumpy lady if I tried this diet, which for the record I wouldn't. Forget the beef—where's the nutrition? Where are there anywhere near the appropriate calories? And where's the chewing? There are certainly some of us who have difficulty chewing and may need softer foods. But, if able, our teeth are there for a reason.

Judith J. Wurtman, PhD, author and founder of the TRIAD weight management center at Harvard Medical School affiliate McLean Hospital, summed it up: "Although a solution of lemon juice and cayenne pepper, if put on the skin, may keep away mosquitoes, it does nothing to support the work of the brain or maintain the integrity of bone mass and muscle strength."

People who go on this diet stay on it anywhere from four to fourteen days. Then they transition to solid food, starting with perhaps vegetable soup, then focusing on fruits and vegetables.

Another cleanse product is the Hollywood Diet. Touted as the "#1 selling detox diet in the country," with over ten million clients, it comes in the twenty-four-hour or forty-eight-hour "Miracle Diet" size. This one hundred-calorie drink is a concoction of juices and botanical extracts. It's fortified with vitamins and minerals. Consumers are told they can lose up to five pounds in twenty-four hours or ten pounds in forty-eight hours. The makers claim many of their customers use the product on a weekly basis. It can then be turned into a meal-replacement diet on their 30-Day Miracle Program plan. The Food and Drug Administration hasn't reviewed the statements made on the product website, so there's also no oversight.

A recent article in *Marie Claire* discussed the "juicerexic." These are rail-thin women who obsessively uses cleanses in order to achieve and maintain super-thin, likely underweight, body frames. That's not a label I'd want pinned on me.

Unfortunately I can't think of one positive thing to say about the cleanse diet. It can cause many side effects, including fatigue, headaches, constipation, diarrhea, and nausea, among other things. McLean Hospital's Wurtman has warned, "The cost can be osteoporosis and frailty, conditions we associate with elderly women confined to wheelchairs." She went on to discuss muscle wasting (aka sarcopenia), which can result from not consuming enough protein coupled with lack of exercise. Symptoms include lack of balance, falls, and frailty.

The UK's National Health Service cautions people not to rely on cleanse diets. Their concerns include:

- *They can cause nutrient deficiencies.*

- *Some herbal ingredients may not be safety tested.*

- *People with certain diseases like diabetes may not be good candidates.*

- *Some cleanse ingredients, such as certain herbs, can adversely affect prescribed medications like birth control pills and Coumadin.*

- *Cleansing may not promote healthy eating in between "detoxes."*

These are all valid issues. One important reason to work with your health care team before going on a VLCD or LCD is to make sure you aren't putting yourself at risk medically.

Fast Times

Fasting has been around for centuries. Certainly many of

us do it for religious reasons. For purposes of weight loss, it goes back as far as Hippocrates, who fasted in order to shed pounds. Recently it has experienced a resurgence. Some plans call for going eighteen to twenty-four hours without eating. Others call for eating food every day, but significantly cutting back calories on several of those days.

Intermittent fasting is one of the new diet plans to hit the scene. It's a huge craze in Britain and Europe, where it's been reported as "the diet of the year." The diet goes by several names, including the fast diet, the Mosley diet, intermittent fasting and the 5:2 diet.

It was introduced across the pond by Michael Mosley, MD, a TV personality who made a documentary, *Eat, Fast and Live Longer*. It aired on the BBC and drew three million viewers, which is considered high ratings there. Dr. Mosley then partnered with writer Mimi Spencer to pen a book on it that was a huge hit. In fact, the *New York Times* reported that in the UK and Britain, "no matter where you go you're likely to hear people around you weighing the pros and cons of famine and feast eating."

The premise is that five days of the week you eat what you want. On the other two days, males restrict their calories to 600 and females to 500 calories for the day. Some diets, like the fast diet, call for the fasting days to be nonconsecutive, while others like the two-day diet, recommend them to be side-by-side.

The diet has also become popular in the United States,

reaching number one on the *New York Times* best-seller hardcover advice and miscellaneous list. It's also been a hit with celebrities, including Beyoncé, Jennifer Lopez, and Ben Affleck.

Proponents of intermittent fasting cite studies linking calorie restriction in mice to a longer lifespan. There's no specific cause identified, but some say reducing calories lowers levels of the hormone IGF-1 (insulin-like growth factor 1). This can lead to protection from heart disease, cancer, and other diseases. Others theorize that intermittent fasting improves the body's sensitivity to insulin.

But there's no definitive study with human subjects that supports the animal research findings. The National Library of Medicine's National Health Service recently found "some evidence that suggests the claims made about it may have some validity—albeit with notable limitations." That's not exactly a resounding endorsement. I'm not a proponent.

Approximately 14 percent of people in the United States have engaged in fasting in order to lose weight.

Can Anyone Spare a Grapefruit?

It never ceases to amaze me how long some of the fad diets have been in existence. Can you believe that the grapefruit diet has been around since the 1930s? Several decades ago it was referred to as the Mayo Clinic diet (not associated with the hospital). This VLCD averages about 800 to 1,000 calories per day. It's a twelve-day program whose followers are told they should lose ten pounds by its completion. But the weight loss is mostly fluid, which isn't lasting.

The meal plan includes, of course, whole grapefruit and unsweetened grapefruit juice, which you eat or drink at each meal. But you can also have a limited amount of other foods, including eggs, bacon and some vegetables. White, yellow, and orange foods are taboo. Fat isn't. As an example, you can have all the butter and salad dressing you want. And you can cook your food however you like, including frying. That's not very heart healthy.

There is some thought among the grapefruit dieters that this vitamin C-rich fruit can burn fat. That's not the case and no scientific evidence points to it. What burns fat? It's tried-and-true physical activity. That's just another reason for us to get moving.

A word here: if you're taking a statin, such as Zocor or Lipitor to lower cholesterol, grapefruit should be off the table. It interacts with the medication in a negative way by accentuating its affects. For questions about other food and drug interactions, I recommend speaking with your health care provider or pharmacist.

Cabbage Soup, It's a Gas!

There are a number of versions of the cruciferous vegetable-based cabbage-soup diet. All of them are very restrictive and very low calorie. The base of the plan is a cabbage soup that has other nonstarchy veggies. It may include bouillon, tomato juice, or onion soup mix. The diet calls for two bowls of soup per day with a limited amount of meat, nonfat and skim milk, and certain fruits and veggies rounding out the day's food allotment. Water is on the menu, but alcohol isn't.

The only positive thing about this diet is there are vegetables in it. It's not healthy or sustainable and the results aren't long-lasting. Connie Diekman, dietitian and director of university nutrition at St. Louis's Washington University, agrees: "It is a monotonous, short-term fix, severely lacking in nutrients, which will result in weight loss that is primarily water and not the essential fat loss that is so important to improving health."

Cotton Ball Baloney

There's actually a diet that includes eating up to five

cotton balls soaked in lemonade, orange juice, or a smoothie as your meal. It's thought that the cotton balls will make you feel full. Some people who follow this diet do eat some food after swallowing the cotton balls. Some don't. This is nothing short of crazy and likely dangerous to your health.

Three for Ten

The 3-Day diet has many names, including the military diet, army diet, navy diet, and more. It has a very strict and specific meal plan for the seventy-two hours in question that weighs in between 800 and 1,200 calories. Oddly, ice cream often appears on the menu, but it's likely still an LCD. Normal eating is resumed after the three day period. Anyway, it promises that you'll lose ten pounds in three days. I'm sure that's long-lasting. Not.

Airy

The breatharian diet would have us believe that we can live on air alone. No food. This diet is insane and not at all advised for someone who wants to live.

Howling at the Moon

The werewolf, or lunar, diet revolves around the lunar

calendar. When the moon is full or new, you fast. Only water and juice are allowed during that time. In response to this diet, the man in the moon must be rolling his eyes.

You Snooze, You Lose

This crazy diet promotes sleeping instead of eating, to the point that it encourages sedatives to keep you snoozing for days. This is nothing short of dangerous. By the way, some say Elvis Presley followed this diet. Look what happened to him.

Bite Marks

Alwin Lewis, MD, who specializes in treating obesity, came up with this diet. You can eat whatever you want, but are only allowed to take five bites of it. If your bites of food are as big as my husband's, perhaps this may work for you. But seriously, this diet is likely too low in calories, and depending on what you choose to eat, could have little in the way of good nutrition.

Hormonal, Anyone?

Not too long ago a menopausal friend of mine told me that she was considering going on the hCG diet. This alarmed me, not only because she was at a healthy weight, but due to the general mechanics of this VLCD. It's calorie restrictive and involves getting either shots of a hormone or the use of serum drops. What hormone? It's the human chorionic gonadotropin, or hCG, which is present in pregnant women's urine. So if you're male or a nonpregnant female, you shouldn't have hCG in your body.

Promoted by the book *The Weight Loss Cure "They" Don't Want You to Know About*, which touts losing thirty pounds in a one-month period, the hCG diet pairs the hormone with an intake of 500 to 800 calories per day. The thought is that hCG works to inhibit hunger and causes our bodies to burn fat for energy. The recommended duration of the diet is forty-five days.

While someone who goes on this diet may lose weight, there's no scientific evidence to suggest it's because of the hCG. Consuming as little as 500 calories a day is the cause. This low calorie intake is almost sure to create nutritional deficiencies. It can also cause an irregular heartbeat and gallstones.

Almost twenty years ago the *British Journal of Clinical Pharmacology* published research that found hCG didn't promote weight loss. More recently, the American Society of Bariatric Physicians didn't recommend hCG as part of a weight-loss plan. Stephen Barrett, MD, director of Quackwatch.org, has described the hCG diet as "extreme, nearly impossible to adhere to, and senseless, especially because the clinical trials have demonstrated that hCG is ineffective as a weight loss aid."

In the United States, the FDA hasn't approved hCG as a weight-loss product. And the FDA and the Federal Trade Commission (FTC) have scrutinized and acted against some companies that sell it for, among other things, falsely promising rapid weight loss.

I'm Starving!

Clearly LCDs and VLCDs aren't all created equal. Some are more questionable than others. But they can all potentially cause side effects and put us at risk for disease. They can also exacerbate existing ones.

It's not uncommon for actors to go on VLCDs in order to lose weight quickly for a movie role. For the film *Dallas Buyers Club*, Matthew McConnaughey lost thirty-eight pounds, about seven pounds per week, by having two egg whites and a Diet Coke in the morning, and then a piece of chicken and another Diet Coke later in the day. That's it. Not surprisingly, he described the diet as difficult and admitted he was "always hungry and irritable."

Taking it a step further, Anne Hathaway said she turned into a "witch" and considers it extraordinary her relationship with her then fiancé, now husband, survived her extreme diet in preparation for her Academy Award-winning role in the movie *Les Miserables*. She lost twenty-five pounds on a VLCD that her costar called "rabbit food." This starvation diet perhaps did more than put her in a bad mood. One of her costars contends that her resulting frailty was the cause of her breaking an arm in a fall.

Ashton Kutcher's health was harmed even more by the VLCD he underwent for his role as Apple cofounder Steve Jobs in the film *Jobs*. For one month he went on a fruitarian diet in which at least 75 percent of calories come from raw fruit. Typically the fruit must have naturally fallen to the ground. Picked fruit is eschewed.

Can we have too much of a good thing? Yes. And Kutcher's diet landed him in the hospital. "I was doubled over in pain, and my pancreas levels were completely out of whack," he recalled. He found the experience "terrifying" considering that Steve Jobs, who died from pancreatic cancer in 2011, was a fruitarian at one point.

Does this mean that we should never embark on a VLCD? I'm not a proponent, but there are varying opinions among health care providers. At a hospital where I worked, they offered LCD and VLCD programs. Their LCD class was a sixteen-week meal-replacement plan. The VLCD was twenty-four weeks long. It was a liquid diet for a full sixteen weeks, then solid food was introduced.

Both the LCD and VLCD programs at this hospital had specific parameters. Participants had to have significant weight to lose. For the VLCD, candidates needed to have a BMI of thirty or above and at least forty pounds to lose. The participants of both diet plans attended a class on nutrition and behavior change each week. They were taught by dietitians, nurses, and lifestyle educators, and covered nutrition, behavior change, and the importance of physical activity. The instructors made sure that when the participants completed the program they had the skills they needed to eat healthily for life.

These patients were medically monitored. To enter into the VLCD class, they got clearance from their doctor, had a recent EKG and lab work, and underwent ongoing monitoring of vitals, among other things. The LCD program members were also monitored. This was done to make sure no one suffered negative consequences. It's the way to do it, if it's done at all. But so many of us don't go that route.

Not everyone is a good candidate for a VLCD, especially:

Children and adolescents

Women who are pregnant or breastfeeding

Type 1 diabetics

People undergoing cancer treatment

Anyone who's had surgery within six weeks of starting the diet

Depending on general health, those fifty and older

People with other conditions

My first teaching foray with a VLCD at a hospital began when I taught the class on week sixteen. This was when the participants started to transition from a liquid diet to solid foods. It's an understatement to say they weren't receptive to the idea. They were practically mutinous. They liked the simplicity of having the liquid product at every meal and they didn't want to let it go. For a while there, I hated life. But they soon warmed to the idea of solid food and everyone went on to incorporate healthy meals into their daily lives.

So you've been on a very restrictive low-calorie diet. And you've lost some weight. But what's next? If you've gone through a medically supervised program, you may have a plan. If you haven't, you might—like so many others before you—creep back to your old habits and gain back all of the weight that you lost so quickly (and perhaps more).

Remember when Oprah lost sixty-seven pounds on a liquid diet? It was in 1988 when she famously went on her show pulling a red wagon that was full of fat equaling the amount of weight that she lost. She proudly wore size-ten jeans. It was quite the visual and left a lasting impression on me. Unfortunately, five years later she'd gained back her lost weight plus twenty-three additional pounds.

As Oprah found, as well as I'm sure some of you have, these types of diets aren't the way to eat for life. They're too restrictive all the way around. That's not a good recipe for long-term weight management.

One of my favorite quotes about restrictive dieting comes from Yoni Freehoff, MD, assistant professor of family medicine at the University of Ottawa and founder and director of its Bariatric Medical Institute. I'm sure many of us can relate when he says, "I sometimes think of blindly restrictive dieting like an icy cold lake on an unseasonably hot day. You work up the nerve to dive in and, after the initial shock wears off and numbness sets in, you splash around happily for a while. But once you climb out, the memory of the initial frigidity is enough to keep you warmly on dry land—diving back in is almost never an option." And you know what? We shouldn't.

SIX

Soup to Nuts

*"From the semi-reasonable to the ridiculous, fad diets make promises
that are simply not sustainable for long-term health."*

—Alexandra Riggle, journalist, *Daily Sundial*

So far we've covered a lot of fad diets. They've all
belonged to a certain type, like gluten-free or high-protein,
low-carb. Some fad diets don't necessarily fall into one
category. Let's now explore some of those.

Typecasting?

These days, some ask "what's my type?" And I'm not
talking about the characteristics that we look for in a
significant other. Think more like a vampire. It's about our

blood type. And by that, I mean O, A, B, and AB. And while I personally have met with very few people who have tried this diet, it's popular and followed by many.

The naturopathic doctor Peter J. D'Adamo believes that our blood type affects our gastrointestinal system and that some foods go better with, or conflict with, certain blood types. He also thinks blood type can influence what diseases we might be susceptible to, and that we should tailor our exercise regime to it. He discusses his ideas in his book *Eat Right 4 Your Type: The Individualized Diet Solution to Staying Healthy, Living Longer & Achieving Your Ideal Weight.*

Naturopathic physicians take a holistic approach to healing through natural therapies and healing practices like nutrition, herbal remedies, and acupuncture. These physicians attend graduate-level naturopathic medical schools for four years. They study the basic sciences that MDs do. In addition, the naturopathic doctor's curriculum includes homeopathic medicine, botanical medicine, clinical nutrition, psychology, and counseling.

Dr. D'Adamo's position is that the various blood types digest lectins (food proteins) differently. He maintains that if you consume lectins that aren't compatible with your blood, it can result in bloating, inflammation, certain diseases like cancer, and a slower metabolism. According to this belief, there are three categories of food:

Highly Beneficial—*considered medicinal*

Neutral

Avoid—*compared to poison*

The premise of the diet is that our blood types evolved during different time periods in history and we should eat accordingly. For example, Dr. D'Adamo believes that type O blood is the oldest and was found in the hunter-gatherers thousands of years ago. Paleo, anyone? Type A came next and appeared when people were getting involved in farming. Type B belonged to the nomads, so a more varied diet works. The youngest blood type, AB, is a combination of its two namesakes. The basics of the diet are:

Blood Type A: *This type is vegetarian. Animal products are excluded. Beneficial foods include grains, organic vegetables, and soy proteins. Gentle exercise is suggested.*

Blood Type B: *Beneficial foods include meat, fruits, vegetables, and low-fat dairy. Lentils wheat and corn are excluded. Moderate exercise is okay.*

Blood Type AB: *Dairy, most produce, tofu, and seafood are beneficial foods. Beef, pork, and chicken are to be avoided. Calming exercise is recommended.*

Blood Type O: *Beneficial foods are fish, poultry, and meat. Foods to avoid include breads, grains, and legumes. Vigorous exercise is okay.*

What can I say about this diet? It just doesn't make sense. First, there's no scientific data to support it. That includes the premise that certain foods and diets are better or worse for specific blood types and that being an O, A, B, or AB is associated with different diseases. There have been no other studies that get the same results as D'Adamo, which is a crucial step. And while the diet doesn't exclude fruits and veggies, which is a good thing, that's about the only positive statement about it I can make.

I love what UK dietitian Juliette Kellow had to say about the "science" behind Dr. D'Adamo's belief on the evolution of blood types: "I'm looking forward to the evolution of blood type F! People with blood type F will need lots of fast food, takeaways, pizza, sugary snacks, crisps, and chocolate to remain in tune with their environment. After all, if the theory is correct, surely that's what we can expect, based on what many of us now eat in the twenty-first century!"

What's That Smell?

I haven't seen any Sensa commercials lately, but for a while there it seemed they were practically constant. I can easily picture the bathing-suit clad actors dancing on the beach to catchy music. Don't we all do that?

Alan Hirsch, MD, the developer of Sensa and founder of Chicago's Smell and Taste Treatment and Research Foundation, says you can eat whatever you want, not have to count calories and still eat less. All it takes is a shake of the wrist. Dr. Hirsch maintains that sprinkling Sensa crystals or "tastants" on your food will do the trick. He claims that you can lose up to thirty pounds in six months while using his product.

Made of tricalcium phosphate, maltodextrin, silica, and flavorings, Sensa comes in a variety of calorie-sodium-and sugar-free flavors. There's one for every taste, including spearmint, cocoa, raspberry, onion, ranch dressing, taco, cheddar cheese, banana strawberry, malt, and horseradish.

Our sense of smell draws us to food. How many of you have responded positively to the wafting vapors of apple pie (or any of your favorite aromatic foods) baking in the oven? I have to say that I'm a sucker for that fresh-baked cookie smell.

And food odor can affect our appetites. Recently, a study by Lorenzo Stafford, MD, saw variations in how thin people and overweight people smell food. The overweight participants in the study were found to pick up food aromas better than the thinner ones. This was more apparent if they'd just eaten. "It could be speculated that for those with a propensity to gain weight, their higher sense of smell for food-related odors might actually play a more active role in food intake," Dr. Stafford said.

Dr. Hirsch uses smell as the basis for the Sensa diet. According to him, the product creates "sensory-specific satiety" to get the smell receptors to tell the brain that we're full.

Does this sound too good to be true? It likely is. The only studies that have been done have been small ones by, you guessed it, Dr. Hirsch himself. There has been no independent research, nor have the Sensa studies been peer-reviewed in medical publications. These are standard for scientific studies. So the data should be questioned. And it has been by me and others. Says Pamela Peeke, MD, "This is not a magic bullet. It oversimplifies the complex physiology and psychology associated with appetite." So be skeptical of this shaker.

And those commercials we haven't seen in a while? The reason may be the FTC recently charged Sensa Products, LLC, its parent company and others with, among other things, deceptive advertising, citing there wasn't "competent and reliable scientific evidence" supporting their claims.

Hills, That Is…Swimming Pools, Movie Stars

Created by the late Judy Mazel, the Beverly Hills diet calls for eating foods in the proper order and combination. For example, fruit and protein aren't to be eaten together. Fruit is meant to be eaten by itself and must be the first thing consumed. Then you can have carbohydrate, followed by protein. You have to wait two hours before eating a different food group. And once you change food groups, you can't go back until the next day.

This doesn't make sense. Order and food combinations don't bring about weight loss. Let's order this diet out the door.

Pucker Up!

There are some who believe that drinking small amounts of vinegar or taking an apple cider vinegar supplement before eating will help with weight loss by curbing appetite and burning fat. But there's only been one study, and that only included one hundred and seventy-five obese people in Japan. These otherwise healthy individuals drank either water or vinegar daily for three months and kept food journals. Those drinking vinegar lost one to two pounds over the twelve-week period. But they gained it all back once the study ended.

And how about what the very acidic vinegar can do to our throats? Mine's burning just thinking about it. And apple cider vinegar can also interfere with certain drugs like insulin and diuretics, as well as some supplements. This can result in low potassium in the body.

Worm Food

I can't believe I'm actually about to discuss a "diet" that involves swallowing a tapeworm. I know, it's ludicrous. But, while probably rare, this practice has been around for quite a while.

In the late nineteenth and early twentieth centuries, there was advertising for "sanitized tapeworms" for females to maintain a trim figure. And it's been purported that opera singer Maria Callas swallowed a tapeworm in an effort to lose weight in the 1950s. It was reported that a tapeworm did find its way into her body, but it's unclear if Callas intentionally orchestrated it. She was known to eat undercooked steak, which is where the tapeworm could have come from. And while she did lose about sixty pounds over several months, it's unlikely that a tapeworm was the direct cause.

In 2013, a woman in Iowa ordered a tapeworm through the Internet and she swallowed it in an effort to lose weight. It didn't work and she had to be treated by a doctor to rid her of the parasite. In essence, she had to be dewormed. "Ingesting tapeworms is extremely risky and can cause a wide range of undesirable side effects, including rare deaths," cautioned the medical director at the Iowa Department of Public Health.

The reality is that a tapeworm doesn't consume enough calories to cause its host to lose significant weight. Malnutrition, anemia, and ascites (fluid buildup in the abdomen) can occur. And if the tapeworm escapes to other parts of your body, it can cause blindness and brain damage. And then there's that pesky problem of death. Enough said.

Ear Stapling

I have to admit that prior to researching this book I hadn't heard of stapling ears for weight loss. That's because it's not an effective tool for shedding pounds and it can lead to ear infection and can even disfigure you.

Based somewhat on the theory of acupuncture, staples are surgically inserted into the inner cartilage of the ears for a couple of weeks or several months. The thought is the staples will affect the pressure point that's associated with regulating appetite, so you eat less and lose weight. It doesn't sound good to me. Pun intended.

The Google Guy's Diet

Ray Kurzweil, leading futurist for Google, is on a diet he thinks could make him immortal. That's right. He may live forever. Forgetting the delusionary and almost certainly wishful thinking by Kurzweil, if it could actually work, are you in? For those of you who say yes, all you need is $1 million a year. That's right. This is the most expensive diet I think that exists today.

What does the diet entail that the cost is so stratospheric? It requires a lot of supplements. Kurzweil takes one hundred pills daily for things like heart, brain, and eye health. Can you imagine that? How long does it take to pop those babies? Who has the time for that? It's way too many pills.

Kurzweil strives to eat healthy meals as well. As an example, his breakfast consists of porridge, berries, smoked salmon and mackerel, dark chocolate with espresso, vanilla soy milk, and green tea. How do I know this? I googled it. You don't have to bother.

Is It Lax?

Some people have turned to laxatives for weight loss. This is considered an abuse of the drug and can be detrimental to health. Laxatives don't stop the absorption of calories. They cause water and electrolyte loss. Electrolytes manage our muscle and nerve function, body hydration, blood pH, and blood pressure. They also regulate the rebuilding of damaged tissue. When our electrolytes are out of whack, we can experience a host of problems, including:

Numbness

Weakness

Fatigue

Twitching

Blood pressure changes

Irregular heartbeat

Seizures

Convulsions

Confusion

Bone disorders

Nervous system disorders

Muscle spasms

Overusing laxatives can result in dependence on them. When the body becomes used to laxatives, it can lead to adverse issues including the inability to have a bowel movement without the drug. It can also cause nausea, vomiting, and diarrhea. Dizziness and fainting can also occur.

Laxatives aren't a good weight-loss tool. If you're currently using them for this purpose, I would advise against it. I recommend that you speak with your doctor regarding it and any symptoms and side effects you may be experiencing.

It's Nuts!

Coconut oil is a saturated fat. Saturated fat isn't good for us. It can make our livers produce too much cholesterol. Raising our cholesterol level may put us at increased risk for heart attacks and stroke.

Sources of saturated fat include:

Whole milk, cream and 2 percent milk

Butter

Ice cream and ice cream products

High-fat cheese

Poultry skin

Beef, lamb, pork, other meats and meat fat
Fully hydrogenated fat
Palm oil
Coconut oil

Yes, coconut oil.

Admittedly borrowing a statement from a fellow dietitian, I like to tell people that coconut oil is good for the skin, but not in the mouth.

The coconut diet combines the high-protein, low-carb diet, the cleanse, and, of course, its namesake, coconut oil, in its weight-loss plan. While coconut oil is a saturated fat, it consists of medium-chain triglycerides, which the body quickly burns. The theory is that it will speed up metabolism and aid in weight loss when added to a low-carb diet.

It also has phases like the diets it embraces. These are:

Phase	Included Foods	Excluded Foods
1	Protein-rich foods like poultry, eggs, cheese, beef, lamb, nuts, eggs, veggies, up to 10 glasses of water, and 2 to 3 tbsp of coconut oil for 21 days.	No carbohydrates, other than nonstarchy veggies.
2 Detox: Kidney, Gallbladder, Liver, or Colon Optional 4-week cleanse	Water with lemon juice and olive oil. Cleansing drinks with vegetables and fiber. Fish, vegetables, and nuts.	May use colonics.
3 Carb Reintroduction	Adds potatoes, whole grains, fruit.	Sugar, alcohol, some fruits, like bananas.
4 Maintenance	Expanded variety of foods.	Sugar, alcohol, some fruits, like bananas.

The 2010 Dietary Guidelines for Americans recommend less than 10 percent of daily calories come from saturated fat. I prefer less than 7 percent of daily calories to be from saturated fat. The less the better.

One tablespoon of coconut oil has 117 calories and 13.6 grams of fat. Of that, 11.764 grams are saturated.

While some recent studies have shown that coconut oil may have a more neutral effect on our cholesterol levels, there isn't conclusive evidence to support this yet. We need to see more studies. Until then, unsaturated fats are the better choice.

The flat-belly diet takes a different approach than the coconut-oil diet. You start with a food restrictive initial four days. Off the plate are processed foods, foods that make you gassy, and certain carbs like bagels, bananas, and pasta. You drink two liters of water mixed with mint leaves, cucumber, lemon, and ginger root daily. After the first four days on the diet, you eat four daily meals of 400 calories each, every four hours. The authors of this diet like the number four. They also like monounsaturated fat and want it eaten at each meal.

Besides the fact that this diet takes some discipline, there's no scientific evidence that suggests a diet can

target a certain area of the body for weight loss.

Who's the Loser?

Whether you watch the show or not, I'm sure the vast majority of us have heard of and know something about the show *The Biggest Loser*. Morbidly obese people undergo very intense diet and exercise regimens to lose weight and vie for the title of "The Biggest Loser."

The show has spawned books and a diet for the masses. It's centered on the 4-3-2-1 Pyramid in which daily food intake includes four servings of vegetables and fruits, three servings of lean protein, two servings of whole grains and 200 extra calories. Eating five to six small meals and drinking six-to-eight glasses of water a day is recommended. Caffeine is a no-no.

Recently Kai Hibbard, one of the 2006 *The Biggest Loser* contestants made the claim that she and other contestants were subject to both physical and emotional abuse. She said they'd get "evil texts" telling them they were going to die without seeing their children grow up and that "fat-person" coffins were ready for them. She talked about contestants being kept prisoner in their hotel rooms and not being able to speak to friends or family. She spoke of her bleeding feet soaking her shoes for the first three weeks of training. "My hair was falling out. My period stopped. I was only sleeping three hours a night," says Hibbard. It sounds awful to me, but I can't say I'm surprised.

In response to Hibbard's claims, NBC said that all contestants are monitored and medically supervised and that the program participants have seen success over the past sixteen show seasons. Regardless of the viewpoint, without the time or trainers, the show's intense (and excessive) exercise schedule is very difficult to translate into daily life. In addition, it's important to be mindful of not consuming less than 1,200 calories. It's a diet that requires extremes and may not be sustainable.

O2 and You

Who doesn't like a diet that promises to make you not only lean, but more beautiful to boot? Say hello to the O2 diet. But can a diet actually make you more handsome or prettier? Not really. Perhaps improved confidence and health from weight loss can bring a spring to our steps, color to our cheeks, a glow to our skin, a sparkle to our eyes, and a sheen to our hair, but overall the diet likely promises unrealistic results.

I find the O2 Diet a bit confusing. It's not based on calories, but on oxygen radical absorbance capacity (ORAC) points. It's all about antioxidants, which can protect us from free radicals in the body that can cause diseases like heart disease and some cancers. I liken antioxidants to police patrolling our bodies that "arrest" the mayhem-causing free radicals and toss them in the clink.

Using the US Department of Agriculture's guide on antioxidant activity of foods, the diet's author, Keri Glassman, RD, claims, "If you eat a diet with a large amount of antioxidants high in ORAC points, you will feel great, look fabulous, be energized and lose weight." Again this sounds great, but it's likely a bit of a tall order.

The diet calls for the follower to reach thirty thousand ORAC points every day. "You can eat all the veggies you want, but you need to pay attention to the portions of fruits, lean proteins, starches, fats, and the indulgences in order to lose weight," says Glassman. She discourages processed foods, fried foods, baked goods, fat-free and sugar-free foods, colas, desserts, added sugars, trans fat, and other high-fat foods.

This diet can be too low in calories and may not include enough protein, grains or dairy products. And according to Lona Sandon, MEd, RD, LD, assistant professor of clinical nutrition at University of Texas Southwestern Medical Center, "There is not enough evidence to use the ORAC scale as a tool for weight loss, because even if a food has a high ORAC value, it may not increase the antioxidant levels or be used by the body to fight free radicals."

Lose the Acid

The alkaline diet is based on pH, a measure of the acidity or base (alkaline) of things. Our body has a slightly alkaline pH of 7.35 to 7.45, while our tummies are solidly in the acid category at a pH of 3.5 or less. It's the acid that helps break down our food.

This diet claims to help keep our body's pH at a good level. But no diet needs to do this. Our body does it for us. Still, the alkaline foods like most fruits, veggies, nuts, seeds, legumes, tofu, and soybeans that it promotes are good for us. This vegetarian diet excludes meat, eggs and dairy, processed foods, most grains, alcohol, and caffeine. So like any vegetarian diet it could lead to some vitamin or mineral deficiency (or both) if we don't eat balanced meals.

WAAAH!

There's actually a diet out there that promotes eating baby food. You know the kind that comes in little jars and requires no chewing. If you have no problems eating solid foods, then I recommend you continue to have foods that you can bite into and chew. You'll be happier, and likely more satisfied, for it.

There's No Magic Pill

We can get OTC weight-loss pills and dietary supplements at a variety of different stores. OTC products aren't subject to the same kind of scrutiny and standards as prescription medications. Many have been found to not be effective. Some can be detrimental to our health. The FDA oversees the safety of these pills and has banned those that can cause us harm, like fenfluramine and dexfenfluramine, which caused heart valve problems. Fenfluramine was one of the ingredients found in the antiobesity prescription drug fen-phen.

Some current OTC diet pills include Alli, green tea extract, guar gum, bitter orange, conjugated linoleic acid, chromium, Hoodia, and chilosan. Of these, so far only Alli has been shown to be effective for weight loss, although not as much as its prescription version, Xenical. But taking it can come with a price in the form of bowel movements that are difficult to control, oily spotting, and loose stools. Not fun. And while rare, it can also injure the liver. That's really not good.

Of the others, guar gum, chromium, chilosan, and bitter orange are probably not effective. Conjugated linoleic acid may be effective for weight loss. We'll see. And there's not enough evidence for Hoodia and green tea extract to draw conclusions. All these products can cause side effects including increased blood pressure and heart rate, constipation, nausea, vomiting, gas, dizziness, nausea, loose stools, diarrhea, vomiting, bloating, abdominal pain, mood changes, headache, and irritability. I'd sure be cranky if I had any one of those.

Here's my second warning about OTCs. Please make sure you let your doctor know about all of the OTC medications you're taking. There's always a risk we might take things that counteract or interfere with prescribed drugs or conditions.

There are also prescription weight-loss drugs available. Some are good for only short-term use, some for the long term. Most of these drugs decrease appetite and increase our sense of being full. These include Lorcaserin (Belviq), Phendimetrazine (Bontril), Phentermine (Suprenza, Adipex), Diethylpropion (Tenuate), Benzphetamine (Didrex), and the combo Phentermine and Topiramate (Qsymia). Orlistat (Xenical) works by blocking fat absorption. All of these drugs can cause side effects, including increased blood pressure and heart rate, dizziness, insomnia, anxiety, nervousness, headache, nausea, dry mouth, intestinal cramping, gas, diarrhea, oily spotting, tingling in the feet and hands, and in the case of Qsymia, birth defects.

In April 2015, Eloise Aimee Shrewsbury, a twenty-one-year-old woman from London, died after taking pills with dinitrophenol (DNP) to aid in losing weight. DNP is an industrial chemical and isn't meant for weight loss, or for that matter human consumption. It's dangerous. Authorities caution anyone from ingesting DNP for any reason.

As far as the cause of Shrewsbury's death, Chief Inspector Jennifer Mattinson released a statement, "The coroner's report will establish the exact cause of Eloise's death, but we urge the public to be incredibly careful when purchasing medicine or supplements over the Internet. Substances from unregistered websites could put your health at risk as they could be extremely harmful, out-of-date or fake." Good advice. So sad for Eloise Aimee Shrewsbury and her family.

Carefully consider the costs and benefits of diet pills. Keep in mind that the pill won't do all of work. We still need to eat sensibly and exercise. This is also crucial once you stop taking the pills. Many people gain back the weight when they do.

It's a Miracle Fruit…Isn't It?

There are also a host of weight-loss supplements out there with a fruit base. Many are touted as miracle weight-loss products. None of them are.

Garcinia cambogia, a pumpkin-shaped fruit, is found in India and Southeast Asia. It contains chlorogenic acid, an active compound said to boost our metabolism, slow the absorption of fat, and prohibit weight gain. People take the rind extract to try and lose weight, but it doesn't appear to be effective. It may help make you feel full with less food, but the studies are mixed and taking it for this use isn't recommended. You can experience side effects such as headaches, nausea, gastrointestinal discomfort, dry mouth, and dizziness. Some people have developed liver problems. Garcinia cambogia also doesn't interact well with certain medications like:

Statins

Iron

Allergy medication (like Singulair and Accolate)

Insulin and pills for blood sugar control

Warfarin

Pain medication

Another fruit, acai berries are small, round, and purple. They're made into products like cleanses and capsules that are promoted for weight loss. Acai berries do contain antioxidants, which are great for health. They fight cell damage from free radicals in our bodies that can cause diseases such as heart disease and cancer. This is fantastic. But there's no evidence that acai berry weight-loss products are effective.

While green coffee beans aren't fruit-based, Dr. Oz caused a stir in 2012 when he discussed using them for weight loss on his TV show. He described the product as "the green coffee bean that burns fat fast." And no exercise needed.

Green coffee beans aren't roasted. Because of this, they contain more chlorogenic acid. So the same premise for weight loss as with Garcinia cambogia is at play here. There haven't been quality studies and the research is preliminary. More studies are needed.

Green coffee beans contain caffeine, which can cause side effects such as increased blood pressure, irregular heartbeat, insomnia, nervousness, restlessness, upset stomach, headaches, and more. In addition, caution should be exercised by pregnant women and those who are nursing, diabetics, and people with bleeding or anxiety disorders, high blood pressure, osteoporosis, diarrhea, irritable bowel syndrome, and glaucoma.

In January 2015, the FTC announced that they'd settled charges against Lindsey Duncan, the maker of the green coffee bean extract and his companies Genesis Today and Pure Health LLC for being deceptive about the product. They claimed that people could lose seventeen pounds and 16 percent of their body fat in twelve weeks, without diet or exercise. They had to pay nine million dollars in refunds to people who bought the coffee bean extract. According to the director of the FTC's Bureau of Consumer Protection, "Lindsey Duncan and his companies made millions by falsely claiming that green coffee bean supplements cause significant and rapid weight loss."

Duncan and company had to stop their weight-loss claims, until two separate clinical studies reach the same results. Apparently, the first study on the green coffee bean extract that was also brought up on *The Dr. Oz Show* was found to be "severely flawed." It should be noted that Dr. Oz didn't know about Duncan's ties to Pure Health at the time of his aired episode.

It's important that appropriate research be conducted on items like weight-loss products. One fruit-based item Dr. Oz discussed on his show several years ago is raspberry ketones—a chemical from red raspberries. He called it a "miracle fat-burner in a bottle." This, of course, caused great interest in using it to lose weight. However, there's no scientific evidence that supports this theory.

There are also no studies regarding safety or potential side effects. But because it's chemically similar to the stimulant synephrine, it's possible that it may cause like side effects including increased blood pressure and rapid heartbeat. It can also cause jitters.

The upshot here is to enjoy fruit for its taste, vitamins, minerals, and health benefits. Choosing fruit over dessert is a great way to lower calorie intake. We don't need to spend our hard-earned money on a fruit-based weight-loss product.

Is the M Plan a Bust?

The M-plan diet, followed by celebs like Katy Perry and Kelly Osbourne, claims that it will help women lose weight. Oddly, it promises that your bust size won't be affected. As we ladies know, one of the first places we lose weight is in our breasts. And let's be honest here—a lot of us want to, at the very least, keep what we have. Some of us would like to lose weight from our hips and thighs and apply some to our two girls. Am I right? And for those of us who'd like to maybe go down a cup size, this is one reason not to attempt this diet.

The diet calls for lunch and dinner to be a mushroom dish only for a two-week period. Mushrooms are loaded with vitamins and minerals like selenium, copper, some of the B vitamins, fiber, and more. They are also low in calories, like all nonstarchy vegetables. So they definitely are a great addition to our diets.

But replacing any meal with vegetables will lower calories consumed in a day. It's not because of the mushrooms. And no diet can target specific areas of the body for weight loss. It would be great if there was, but sadly there isn't.

It's in the Mail

Jenny Craig, Nutrisystem, and the like are programs in which you buy prepackaged meals and snacks from the company. It's convenient, portion controlled, and balanced. Calorically they're fairly reasonable, although they can be too low for some. As an example, females get a 1,200 calorie plan and males a 1,500 calorie plan on Nutrisystem. Jenny Craig counselors work with the individual to determine calorie needs. The only thinking, shopping, and preparation you have to do is adding in fruits, vegetables, whole grains, and low-fat and nonfat dairy.

Jenny Craig, a division of Nestle, has two programs. One is for those of us who prefer to handle everything from the comfort of our homes. Phone, mail, and the Internet are the communication and information channels. But Jenny also has centers. In the United States and Canada there are four hundred and ninety-seven of them. Jenny Craig also has a presence in Australia, New Zealand, and France. Members can have weekly face-to-face meetings with their counselors. Nutrisystem is primarily online.

The following is a comparison of the two programs:

	Nutrisystem	Jenny Craig
Cost	Free to join. Food cost depends on your individual plan, but it's approximately $260 to $550 or more per month. Counseling and other tools are free.	On the high side. There's an upfront $99 enrollment fee. Food can cost about $500 to $700 or more per month.
Food/Meals	Offers diabetic, gender specific, vegetarian, and other individually specific plans.	Has vegetarian, frozen, and shelf-stable foods.

	Nutrisystem	Jenny Craig
Dining Out	Eating out is fine, but the meal should be low in calories and fat.	Jenny's rules need to be followed when dining in restaurants.
Physical Activity	At least 30 minutes a day is recommended. Members receive a CD and there are online physical activity plans for yoga, aerobics, and resistance training.	Exercise is encouraged, but no specific plans are offered.
Support	There's a large online community.	You can access online message boards and chat rooms. The main communication is through the counselors.
Counseling	Support is available around the clock, seven days a week. You can communicate by phone (toll free) or e-mail. Counselors may be dietitians, diabetes educators and other healthcare professionals.	Counselors are registered dietitians and psychologists. You can speak and meet with them weekly.

	Nutrisystem	Jenny Craig
Pros	• Great variety of foods • Food delivery • 24/7 online support with online classes, behavior modification guides and self-monitoring tools. It syncs with Apple Health, Jawbone, Fitbit and others.	• Specials available for new members • Physical centers • Weekly progress meetings with counselors and online articles, recipes and a mobile app. • Counselors work to wean members off
Cons	• Cost • Keeping weight off after you quit the program may be difficult.	• Expensive food and has a joining fee.

There are also food delivery plans that are less packaged and fresher fare, such as Seattle Sutton's Healthy Eating. But like all the meal programs, what happens when you're finished with it and ready to strike out on your own? What skills have you learned to shop, cook, make better choices, and more? It can leave us lacking.

Where to Go, What to Do?

We've now covered a lot of the diets that are out there. Is your head spinning? Are you questioning which path is best to take? Read on. The answers lie ahead.

LISA TILLINGER JOHANSEN

PART TWO

THE PLAN

LISA TILLINGER JOHANSEN

SEVEN

Keep It Simple...Smarty!

"What's more simple than a plate?"

—First Lady Michelle Obama

We've talked about a lot of diets so far. It's amazing how many there are. And new ones are introduced all the time. Let's be honest here, some of them are downright nutty. Others not quite as much. There are likely still a few that you might be on the fence about them. Climb over, pardner and walk away into the setting sun.

Because what's the takeaway here? Fad diets aren't good. They're not a long-term plan and they can be detrimental to our health. Let's make a pact to just say no to them. Are you in? Good.

I did touch on a few diets like the Mediterranean, DASH and the reversal. These aren't considered fad diets and are fine to follow. And there are a few more like Volumetrics and Weight Watchers that are worth looking at. I'll talk about them in the chapters to come. They all have a commonality to them that we can pull together and simplify. Easy is best.

Many think of the word *diet* in a negative way. I prefer a positive approach and like to talk about a healthy eating plan for life. This is something that once we embark on it, we're in for the long term. It's the last and best "diet" we'll be on. So where do we begin? Let's start with the plate.

A Plate, Not a Platter

The confusing food guide pyramid has bitten the dust. It served as our dutiful meal planning navigator for many years, but a less convoluted symbol has taken its place. We now look at the healthy plate. The USDA has its version and a comprehensive website about it at choosemyplate.gov. Here's what their recommended plate looks like:

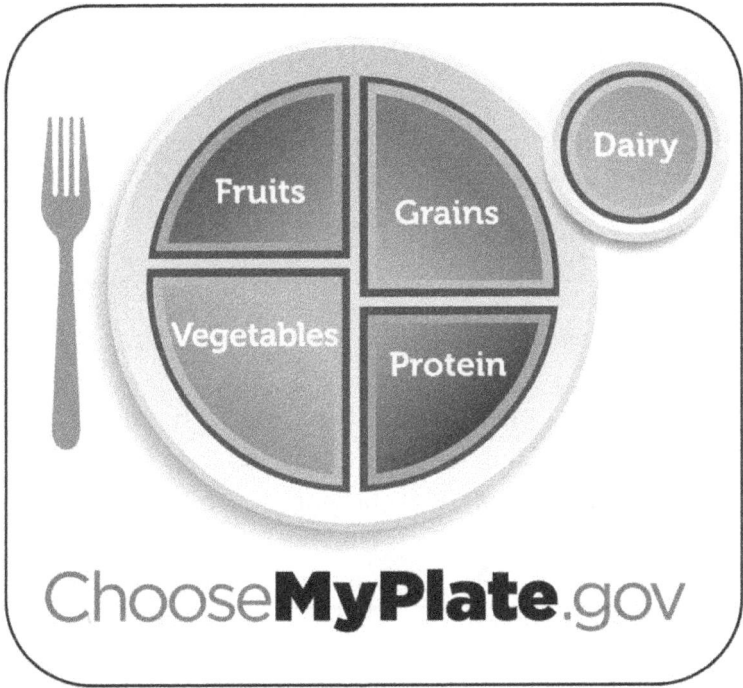

ChooseMyPlate.gov

This is a great way to lay out your meal. So if it looks good to you, go for it. I've been suggesting a slight variation of this plate model for years. And by *plate*, I mean just that. I don't mean a platter. We're looking at a nine-inch one, which is a small. Many restaurant plates are bigger than nine inches. Mine at home, as I'm sure is true for most of us, are twelve inches. If you find yourself with a twelve-inch plate in your hand, do what I tell my clients to do. Mentally cut it back a bit and don't fill it to the rim.

The version I use calls for half the plate to be nonstarchy vegetables, a quarter to be starch, and the other quarter to be lean protein. Fruit and nonfat or low-fat dairy are outside the plate. When I draw it on the board for my clients to see, it looks like Mickey Mouse's head, with fruit in one ear and low-fat or nonfat dairy in the other. It's so simple and easy to remember. After all, it's the happiest plate…on the table.

I know this goes without saying, but don't build mountains of food in the allotted spaces on the plate. This will definitely defeat the point.

So what's the reasoning behind the portioning of the plate? Why's it balanced the way it is? Let's take a look.

I'll Take Half

Half the plate is nonstarchy veggies. But not everyone knows what those are. For example, many people tell me they think the much-maligned carrot is a starchy vegetable. But it's not. It's nonstarchy. Because there are so many more nonstarchy veggies than starchy ones, I always give my clients the much shorter list of the starchy veggies. These should only take up a quarter of the plate. They are:

Beans

Cassava

Corn

Parsnips

Peas

Plantains

Potato (of all color, and yes I mean sweet potatoes and yams)

Winter squash

It's important to prepare all foods in a healthy manner, even nonstarchy veggies like spinach, broccoli, tomatoes, carrots, cabbage, green beans, and asparagus. It's certainly possible to take something naturally low in calories and fat and make it less healthy by the way we prepare it.

I'm from Georgia and we southerners like to fry everything. Even pickles. But if I fill my plate with fried okra, I'm not doing well by myself. I might as well just eat a donut. Steaming, microwaving, baking, broiling, and raw are all good ways to prepare vegetables. Avoid sauces and limit oil or butter (trans fat-free margarines are okay). But remember that a serving size of oil, butter, or trans fat-free margarine is one teaspoon.

I like my vegetables as they come in nature, plain and delicious. For measurement purposes, one cup of raw veggies or a half cup of cooked is a serving size.

A 2013 Swedish study that followed more than seventy-one thousand people age forty-five to eighty-three for thirteen years found that those who didn't eat fruits and vegetables died on average three years earlier than those who did. At least five servings of fruits and veggies a day was found best for optimum health.

Nature's Multivitamins

Often when I teach a nutrition class, I'll hand out fruits and vegetables to the attendees. Instead of calling them by their names, I'll say "let's eat some health." They're that good for us. That's why we can make half our plate nonstarchy veggies and include a fruit outside the plate.

Vitamins, minerals, and antioxidants abound in fruits and veggies. Antioxidants can protect our cells from the damage causing free radicals—molecules created when the body breaks down food or from exposure to environmental toxins like radiation and tobacco smoke. These dangerous molecules can damage our cells, which can lead to cancer, heart disease, and other diseases and conditions. Antioxidants are our warriors who battle this. Sources include:

Beta-carotene

Lutein

Lycopene

Selenium

Vitamins A, C, and E

Foods with antioxidants include veggies, fruits, grains, nuts, and some poultry, fish, and meats. The color of our food can also clue us in to their health properties. I tell people to eat their colors as the hue is important. Let's see:

- **White:** *White fruits and veggies contain anthoxanthins, a polyphenol compound that contains antioxidants. They can lower the risk of cancer and heart disease. Some white foods, like garlic, have allicin, which can lower the risk for high cholesterol, high blood pressure, heart disease, and cancer. White foods can be good sources of vitamin C, potassium, riboflavin, folate, and niacin. A November 2011 study found that consuming white veggies and fruits can reduce the risk of stroke.*

- **Yellow and Orange:** *Carotenoids give fruits and veggies these colors. They can reduce the risk for vision problems, cancer, and heart disease, as well as improve the immune system. Yellow and orange fruit and veggies can contain folate, bromium, vitamin C and potassium. The body converts the carotenoid Beta-carotene into vitamin A.*

- **Purple, Blue, and Red:** *Purple, blue and red fruit and veggies contain anthocyanins, which have antioxidant properties and can reduce the risk for stroke, heart disease, degeneration of the eyes, and memory issues. Red fruits and veggies also often have lycopene, which can lower the risk for heart disease and cancer. Compounds in red, blue, and purple fruit and veggies can also reduce the risk for urinary tract infections, and can help maintain healthy vision and a good immune function.*

- **Green:** *The color is due to chlorophyll. Some green fruits and veggies also have indoles, which can reduce cancer risk. They may also contain lutein, which can help vision. Other nutrients often present in green veggies and fruits include vitamins A, C, and K and folate.*

Fabulous Fiber

A hidden gem in foods is fiber. It's found in whole grains, vegetables, fruits, split peas, lentils, and cooked beans. It's the part of the plant that we don't digest and it can do so much for us. Besides helping to keep us regular, manage blood sugar, lower cholesterol, prevent constipation, potentially decrease colon cancer risk, and manage diverticulosis and irritable bowel syndrome, it can help keep us full. This can be instrumental when we're trying to manage our weight. By replacing foods low in fiber with higher fiber choices, we'll likely eat less.

There are two types of fiber, soluble and insoluble.

Soluble fiber dissolves in water and insoluble fiber doesn't. Insoluble fiber helps prevent constipation and is good for our digestive tract. It's found in grains, breads, cereals, fruits, veggies, nuts, seeds, and popcorn. Soluble fiber can help manage blood sugar and lower cholesterol. Sources include rye, barley, rice, bran, oats, legumes, ground flaxseed, psyllium, and fruit.

There are some whole-grain white breads, so they have more fiber. These are made from 100 percent whole-wheat flour that's white. Conversely, some brown breads can have that color because caramel is an ingredient, but 100 percent whole wheat isn't. And it should be. So read the food labels.

If you're confused about grain jargon, see below:

- **Refined:** *The bran and germ of the grain kernel are removed during processing.*

- **Processed Food:** *A food that's been treated to alter its chemical, physical, sensory, or microbiological properties.*

- **Whole Grain:** *A grain that's been completely milled, but not refined.*

- **Enriched:** *The addition of nutrients lost through processing. This often includes folate, niacin, iron, riboflavin, and thiamin.*

• **Fortified:** *The addition of nutrients to a food that weren't originally contained in the food, or was only present in small amounts.*

Aim for twenty-one to thirty-eight grams of fiber a day. This may sound hard for some, considering that recent studies have shown that the average person in the United States gets approximately fourteen to fifteen grams a day. But if you make better choices, the gram count will add up fast.

Tips to Increase Fiber Intake

- *Eat five or more servings of fruits or vegetables each day.*
- *Limit, or better yet, avoid fruit juice.*
- *Eat the edible seeds and skin of fruits and vegetables.*
- *Enjoy fruit for dessert instead of cake, pie, or ice cream.*
- *Eat split peas, lentils, and cooked beans often.*
- *Put no-salt-added canned beans in casseroles, soups, and salads.*
- *Have six to eleven servings of cereal, rice, pasta, and whole-grain breads a day.*
- *Look for cereals and breads that list 100 percent rye, corn, or whole wheat as the first ingredient on the nutrition facts label.*
- *Choose popcorn, quinoa, brown rice, bran cereals, oats and bran, whole-wheat tortillas and pastas.*
- *Add unprocessed wheat bran to soups, cereals, casseroles, and more.*

• *Limit refined grains such as white rice, white bread, pretzels, enriched pasta, and saltine crackers.*

If you're not eating a lot of fiber now, don't double your intake overnight. You'll pay a gassy and bloated price. Add fiber slowly and drink water.

The First Quarter

The quarter of the plate occupied by your protein source should also be a healthy choice. Fish, poultry (no skin), eggs (I limit egg yolks), lentils, beans, nuts, or tofu are recommended. If you eat red meat, the gold standard is to only have it once or twice a month and to choose leaner cuts. As with the veggies, baking, broiling, grilling, and roasting are examples of healthy methods of food preparation.

If I told my husband he could never have red meat, or even eat it just twice a month, he might cry. So keep in mind that any change is good. Small steps lead to big changes. For example, if you're eating red meat three times a week, try cutting back to once or twice a week. While you should work on cutting back some more over time, you're still better off with any reduction in consumption.

Our bodies use protein to help us maintain our normal body functions and keep our organs and muscles in tip-top shape. It also helps us to build and replace hair, blood, and muscles. One gram of protein equals four calories.

One quarter of the plate is equal to about three ounces of protein. I mentioned this earlier, this doesn't mean that we should have nine ounces of meat, fish, poultry, etc., each day. I recommend about an ounce for breakfast and two to three ounces each for lunch and dinner. One ounce of protein equals one whole egg, two egg whites, or one piece of string cheese.

Besides being one quarter of the plate, you can also gauge portion size of protein by eyeballing it. Three ounces should be about the size of your palm (not the whole hand), a deck of cards or a cassette tape. If you're at home and have a scale handy, you can always weigh it. Remember, lean proteins are the way to go. If there's a lot of fat, or marbling, trim it off. Or look elsewhere. And don't forget to remove the poultry skin.

The Second Quarter

The remaining quarter of the plate is for starchy veggies and grains such as pasta, rice, corn, peas, beans, potatoes, a slice of whole-grain bread, or one six-inch whole wheat or corn tortilla. Half of our grain servings each day should be of the whole variety. Choose those that have at least three grams or more of fiber per serving. (When eating breakfast cereals, aim for at least five grams or more of fiber in one serving.) Whole grains aren't as processed and contain more vitamins, minerals, and fiber than their more refined counterparts. They are typically brown in color, not white. Be sure to look for the word *whole*. If it doesn't say it, you're probably not getting enough bang for your fiber buck.

Studies show that those of us who eat mostly unprocessed carbs (legumes, whole grains, fruit, veggies) have a lower rate of obesity, heart disease, cancer, and diabetes. But the average person in the United States eats more processed carbs than we did thirty years ago. This equates to thirty-five pounds more white flour and thirty pounds more sugar.

A word about carbohydrates. Carbs are all grains (rice, pasta, bread, crackers, cereal, etc.), starchy veggies, sugar, jam, jelly, pie, cookies, and other sweets. There are carbohydrates in milk and yogurt as well. Fruit is also a carb. Just about everything but proteins and fats are in this group.

We use carbohydrates as our main energy sources. About 50 percent, or a little less, of our calories should come from them. One gram of carbohydrate equals four calories.

Contrary to what some say, carbohydrates don't make us fat. Good choices and quantity matter, though. Complex carbs (unrefined) gives a slow and steady energy source. They're not as likely to be converted to fat.

Ear One

With dairy, we're now off of that nine-inch plate and into one of the ears. Dairy products provide a lot of good things for us, not the least of which is calcium. Aim for low-fat and nonfat sources (whole milk is usually only for those who are two and younger). Two to three servings of dairy a day is recommended (unless you have certain conditions like kidney disease in which dairy should be limited). A serving size is eight ounces of milk or plain yogurt, or six ounces of fruited yogurt. A serving size of cheese is one ounce.

I recommend that you measure the amount of liquid your beverage glasses hold. They can contain a lot more than you may think. I recently taught a series of weight management classes in which one of the participants kept an online food diary on myfitnesspal.com. He drank several glasses of 1 percent milk every day and would input two eight-ounce glasses into his diary. About nine weeks into the twelve-week series, he finally measured the liquid volume the glass held. It wasn't eight ounces. It was sixteen ounces. Ouch.

If you're lactose intolerant, there are milk products out there for you. Lactose is a sugar present in milk and milk products such as ice cream, pudding, processed cheese and cheese sauce, smoothies, cream soups, milk chocolate, and milk shakes. These items can cause cramping, bloating, and diarrhea in those who are lactose intolerant.

Foods that are low in lactose include yogurt, natural cheese, butter, sherbet, and cottage cheese. Lactose-free milk like Lactaid, calcium-fortified soy milk, almond milk, and rice milk are good choices for anyone who's lactose intolerant. Soy yogurt, calcium-fortified soy cheese, and soy frozen desserts are good too.

Good sources of nondairy calcium include tofu made with calcium, cooked turnip greens, broccoli, kale, spinach, sardines, canned salmon with bones, dried figs, and calcium-fortified foods.

Ear Two

We place fruit on the other ear. Fruit tastes good and benefits us. I recommend whole and cut fruit (fresh, canned in its own juice, or frozen) over juice. Two to four servings a day is suggested. A serving size is equal to one small-to-medium piece of whole fruit, one cup of mixed berries, half a banana, or a quarter of melon such as cantaloupe.

A serving size of juice is four ounces or half a cup. Is that the amount you drink? Most of us who enjoy juice tend to gulp down way more than that. And if it's the fruit variety, then we're consuming too many calories. I've seen single-size bottles of this sweet beverage that contain 240 calories plus. And I'm not talking about a smoothie that can have 800 calories or more. It's not the best choice. Also, it takes no time at all to swig a serving of fruit juice.

Eating the whole fruit is the better choice. It typically has less calories and it takes longer to eat fruit than it does to drink its juice. This is good because it takes twenty minutes for the stomach to tell the brain it's full. This makes slower eating better. And fruit juice typically isn't a good fiber source unlike its solid counterpart.

Fat Joins In

While fat doesn't have its own spot on the plate, a small amount, one to two servings, may be included at each meal.

And I mean small. A serving size of oil is one teaspoon. One tablespoon of regular dressing or two tablespoons of reduced fat dressing is considered a serving size.

I never fail to get gasps of shock and dismay when I hold up the food model of a serving size of avocado. It's one-eighth of the avocado or two level tablespoons. Believe it or not, this small amount is forty-five calories.

A great way to estimate a serving size of nuts (a protein and a fat) is to put the nuts in one of your hands and close that hand comfortably making a fist. You aren't holding the fist shut with your other hand and nuts aren't falling out the sides. That's a serving size. This is equivalent to six almonds or cashews, ten peanuts, sixteen pistachios, four walnut halves, or two Brazil nuts.

Fats give us energy. But they're very high in calories and need to be limited. One gram of fat equals nine calories, over double the amount found in a gram of protein or carbohydrate.

There are four types of fat: monounsaturated, polyunsaturated, saturated, and trans fat. I'm invariably asked about the "heart-healthy" ones. Monounsaturated fats are the best choices. They include olive, canola and peanut oil, avocado, most nuts, nut butters, seeds, and olives. These fats can lower total cholesterol, improve HDL (good cholesterol), and reduce the risk of heart disease.

Polyunsaturated fats include the heart-healthy omega-3 fatty acids. These can help lower triglycerides, reduce the risk of blood clot formation, and prevent and treat heart disease. They can also raise HDL. Good sources of omega-3 fatty acids include flaxseed and flaxseed oil, walnuts, and fatty fish like mackerel, trout, salmon, albacore tuna, and sardines. Non-omega-3-containing polyunsaturated fats can lower LDL (bad cholesterol) and can reduce heart disease risk. Sources are cottonseed, grapeseed, safflower, soybean, and corn oils.

One fat to limit or avoid is saturated fat. It can raise total cholesterol and increase the risk of heart disease and stroke. As previously mentioned, saturated fats include beef, lamb, pork, and other meats, meat fat, poultry skin, palm oil, coconut oil, and whole and 2 percent milk and milk products.

The other fat to stay away from is trans fat. This is a fat that can occur naturally in some foods, but is often made through processing to increase the shelf life of foods. Sources include margarine, baked goods such as cookies, crackers, and biscuits, as well as fried foods like donuts. Trans fat can raise LDL and triglycerides, lower HDL and increase the risk of getting diabetes. It's so bad that as of June 2015, the FDA is requiring partially hydrogenated oil (trans fat) to be phased out of processed foods over the next three years.

In addition to more carbohydrate intake, many Americans eat and drink much more fat today than we did thirty years ago. We consume fourteen more pounds of cheese, twenty more pounds of meat, and twelve more pounds of fat annually.

Go easy on the fat. Small portions still pack a caloric punch.

It's All in the Plate

So given everything we've learned about the healthy plate method and the contributions the food groups make to our overall body function and health, I hope you see that this eating plan is a common-sense approach. It's certainly easy. It does the trick.

LISA TILLINGER JOHANSEN

EIGHT

Size Matters

"Over the past few decades portion sizes of everything from muffins to sandwiches have grown considerably. Unfortunately, America's waistbands have reacted accordingly."

—Liz Monte, lifestyle contributor for divinecaroline.com

If we stay within the parameters of the healthy plate, lay it out as we should, prepare our food in a healthy manner, and don't build the great pyramid with our portions, we're on the right path. But I think it's a good idea to expand our knowledge a bit. The more we know, the better off we are. And in the case of our food, one of the areas where we veer off is in portion sizes. Bigger isn't better.

Do you think you serve yourself up appropriate portion sizes? That's the $64,000 question. This is a topic that warrants discussion.

Measurements Don't Lie

It's not uncommon for many of us to overeat. I've given you a "taste" of recommended serving sizes and some of it may have been surprising. Quantity does matter. If we put too much of even a good thing in our mouth, we may pay for it on the scale.

There's a difference between serving size and portion size. Serving size is the recommended amount we should eat. Portion size is what we actually serve ourselves. Do you think the amount you eat equals the item's serving size? Let's find out.

Here's a more comprehensive look at what are considered serving sizes:

Starch*

- **Bread (white, whole wheat, etc.):** 1 slice of sandwich bread
- **Crackers (round and saltine-type):** 6
- **English Muffin:** 1/2
- **Hamburger/Hot Dog bun:** 1/2
- **Oatmeal:** 1/2 cup
- **Pancake/Waffle:** 1 (4-inch)
- **Pasta:** 1/2 cup
- **Pita Bread:** 1/2 six-inch in width
- **Polenta, Quinoa, Rice (white, brown), Barley, Couscous:** 1/2 cup (1/3 cup for diabetics)
- **Popcorn:** 3 cups
- **Stuffing:** 1/3 cup
- **Taco Shell:** 2, each 5 inches in width
- **Tortilla (corn, flour):** 1, 6 inches in diameter (a 10-inch tortilla is three servings)

Starchy Vegetables, Beans, Lentils, Peas

- **Beans (all but green beans), peas, and lentils:** 1/2 cup, 1/3 cup baked beans for diabetics
- **Cassava (yucca):** 1/2 cup
- **Corn:** 1/2 of the cob or 1/2 cup
- **Plantains:** 1/2 cup
- **Potato (boiled, mashed), including yams:** 1/2 cup mashed, baked—3 oz
- **Pumpkin (unsweetened, canned):** 1 cup

- **Winter squash:** 1 cup

Fruit

- **Apple:** 1 (4-oz)
- **Banana:** 1 small (4 oz) or half of one medium or large
- **Blueberries:** 3/4 cup
- **Canned fruit:** 1/2 cup
- **Dried fruit (raisins, cranberries, etc.):** 2 level tbsp
- **Dates, prunes:** 3
- **Fruit cup:** 1/2 cup
- **Grapefruit:** 1/2 of whole or 3/4 cup of sections
- **Grapes:** 17 small or 10–11 medium to large
- **Orange:** 1 (6 1/2 oz)
- **Strawberries:** 1 1/4 cup whole berries
- **Watermelon:** 1 1/4 cup cubed

Nonstarchy Vegetables

- **Includes all vegetables except the starchy ones, which are corn, peas, beans, parsnips, plantains, potato, and pumpkin:** 1 cup raw or 1/2 cup cooked

Dairy

- **Milk (all types but evaporated):** 1 cup
- **Yogurt:** 1 cup plain or 3/4 cup fruited

Protein

- **Meat, fish, poultry, eggs, cheese, etc.:** 2 to 3 oz for lunch and dinner, 1 oz for breakfast (1 oz equals 1 whole egg, 2 egg whites, 1 piece of string cheese)

*With regard to starch, 3 to 4 servings of starch per meal isn't excessive. So, for example, if you have a turkey sandwich with two slices of whole wheat bread, a piece of fruit, salad greens, and a glass of nonfat milk, you're having approximately 4 servings of carbohydrates.

Another way to gauge recommended serving sizes is by equating them to common items. Let's take a look:

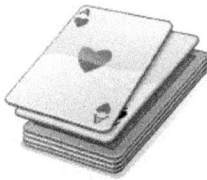

A deck of cards equals approximately 3 ounces of meat, poultry, or fish.

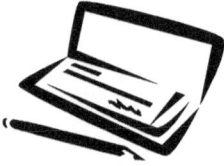

A checkbook is about the size of 3 ounces of fish.

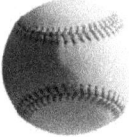

A baseball is approximately the size of 1 cup of cold cereal, a cup of salad greens, or 1 medium piece of fruit. Half of the baseball equals 1/2 cup of ice cream, 1/2 cup of fruit, 1/2 cup of cooked pasta or rice, and a serving size of potato.

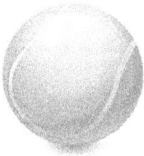

A tennis ball equals about the size of 1 cup of cooked pasta or rice, one serving of whole fruit or 15 grapes.

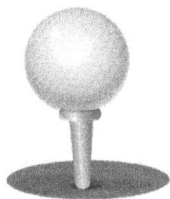

A golf ball (or ping pong ball) is approximately the size of 2 tablespoons of peanut butter.

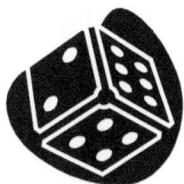

One die equals about 1 teaspoon of peanut butter, margarine, or other spreads. Four stacked dice are approximately the size of 1.5 ounces of cheese or 2 slices of cheese.

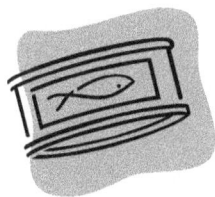

A 6-ounce can of tuna is approximately the serving size of a bagel or a roll.

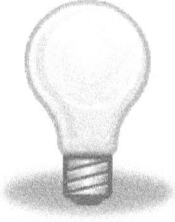

A light bulb equals 1 cup of raw veggies.

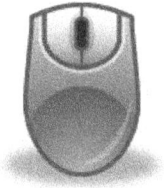

A computer mouse is approximately the size of a medium potato.

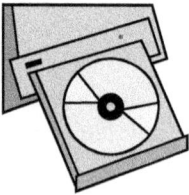

One CD is the same size as a serving of a pancake.

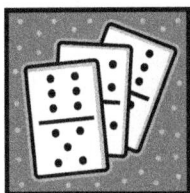

Three dominos equal 1.5 to 2 ounces of cheese.

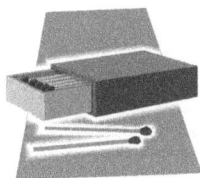

A matchbox is approximately the size of 1 ounce of meat or 1 tablespoon of salad dressing, oil, or mayonnaise.

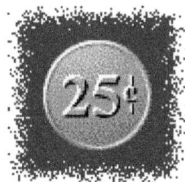

A quarter in diameter equals about 1 teaspoon of oil.

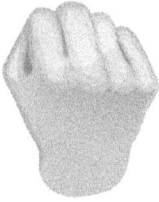

A fist is about the size of 1 cup. It also equals the serving size of 1 baked potato. And if you place nuts inside that closed fist, you'll have portioned out an appropriate serving.

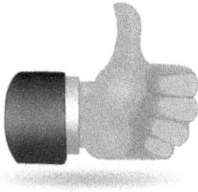

A thumb equals approximately 1 tablespoon or 1 ounce of cheese. The tip of the thumb is equivalent to a teaspoon.

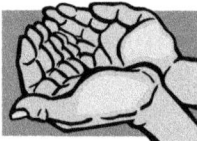

Two cupped hands can be a serving size of chips. One open handful equals about 1 cup or 1 to 2 ounces of snack food.

The Excess of Our Lives

There are many countries in the world where restaurants, theaters, etc., serve proper portion sizes. The United States isn't one of them. Let's take a look at portion sizes in America and how that compares to recommended serving sizes.

Item	Portion Sizes	One Recommended Serving Size	Calories in Served Portion vs. Calories in One Recommended Serving	Fat Grams in Served Portion vs. One Recommended Serving
Bagel	4 ounces	1.5 ounces	320 vs. 120 (2 tablespoons of cream cheese adds an additional 100 calories and 10 grams of fat.)	3 grams vs. 1 gram
Chocolate Chip Cookie	5 ounces	1 ounce	700 vs. 140	20 grams vs. 4 grams

Item	Portion Sizes	One Recommended Serving Size	Calories in Served Portion vs. Calories in One Recommended Serving	Fat Grams in Served Portion vs. One Recommended Serving
Pepperoni Pizza	4 slices of a 14-inch pizza with a total of 12 slices.	2 slices of a 14-inch pizza with a total of 12 slices.	920 vs. 460	36 grams vs. 18 grams
Tortilla Chips	40	10	400 vs. 100	20 grams vs. 5 grams

Most sit-down restaurants in the United States serve giant portions. I embarrass my husband to no end by often carrying a scale and measuring cups and spoons with me when we go out to eat. I find it very interesting and helpful. For example, the Italian restaurants we've visited, from mom-and-pops to chains, typically give us between two and four cups of pasta in one entrée. A serving size should be half a cup for nondiabetics and a third of a cup for diabetics.

And did you know that one ladle provided at the crocks of dressing at salad bars typically holds three tablespoons? A serving size is one tablespoon of regular dressing and two tablespoons of the nonfat versions. And I've seen people ladle and ladle and ladle high-calorie dressings onto their salads. I'm sure many of them think they're eating a nutritious meal. But the calorie count of all that dressing is off the charts.

Sandwiches and burgers also break the calorie scale. I've weighed the meat patty from my husband's hamburger on numerous occasions and some of them have been as large as twelve to thirteen ounces. That's a lot more than the recommended three ounces. And what about a deli sandwich? I don't know how people can eat them as is. I can't even open my mouth wide enough to get my mouth around one and take a bite. They're crazy big.

I could go on and on, but I'm sure your get the message. Just about every menu item is suspect as far as serving sizes go, so look at them with a discerning eye.

But since the majority of our meals are eaten at home, it's also important to pay attention there. Are you following the healthy plate? How about consuming the recommended serving sizes? Do you prepare your food in a healthy manner? Definitely food for thought.

I challenge my clients to determine the quantity of what they've been eating. A question I always ask is how they pour cereal into their bowls. How do you? Do you take the box and pour into the bowl until it looks good? Next

time you go to eat cereal, I suggest you pour the cereal into your bowl like you usually do. Then before you put in the milk, take a measuring cup and see how much you've put in the bowl. It may be more than a serving size. Do this for other foods such as rice, pasta, and more.

What would eating the following day's worth of meals with today's serving sizes compared to those from twenty years ago mean calorically? Let's see:

The Meal

• **Breakfast :** *A 6-inch bagel and a 16-ounce coffee with milk and sugar*

• **Lunch :** *2 slices of pepperoni pizza and a 20-ounce soda*

• **Dinner:** *Chicken Caesar salad and a 20-ounce soda*

Okay, there are definitely some less healthy choices in the above meal, like the large regular sodas, but even given that, it's astounding to think that this day's worth of meals would have 1,595 more calories today than two decades ago. That's how much serving sizes have grown over the years. And, if we ate this same meal every day for a year, we'd add on over 500,000 additional calories. Wow.

Knowing recommended serving sizes and determining your portion sizes is essential. The two may be quite different. But knowledge is power and with regard to serving sizes versus portion sizes, the more you know about how much you're eating will help you determine where you can make changes. You can't go wrong there.

LISA TILLINGER JOHANSEN

NINE

Drink Up!

"It's all right to drink like a fish—if you drink what a fish drinks."

—Author Mary Pettibone Poole

We don't just include food in our diets. We also drink beverages. If you're like me, you always have a glass, cup, or bottle nearby. What's my poison? It's decaf hot tea. I love it. I can't get enough.

Whatever we like, we all drink some form of liquids. From water, to juice, to soda, coffee, vino, and more, we enjoy beverages daily. That's a good thing, because beverages are essential to our health. Or they can be detrimental. Like food, good choices matter when choosing our liquid refreshments. Many of us don't think about what our beverages contain. Calories, fat, caffeine, etc. all matter.

Talk About Drought

Our bodies need fluids. They keep us hydrated, which is important. Remember, our bodies are about 60 percent water. We don't do well when our levels are low.

We experience dehydration when we lose more fluids than we take in. When this happens, our bodies don't have sufficient water and other fluids to maintain normal functions. Causes of dehydration include:

Vomiting

Severe diarrhea

Fever

Excessive sweating

Not drinking enough water when the weather's hot or during exercise

People of all ages can become dehydrated, but young kids and older adults are at highest risk. So are people with chronic disease. Mild to moderate dehydration can usually be treated by consuming more fluids. But severe cases require quick medical treatment.

I work extensively with older adults and am always encouraging them to drink fluids, preferably water. Many of them don't have at least five beverages a day, even on scorching hot summer days. Some have experienced difficulties, including hospitalization, for failure to drink enough liquids.

In addition to keeping us hydrated, fluids help remove toxins for our bodies. They're good for our muscles, moisten our tissues, and cushion our joints. They bring nutrients to our cells. Fluids help keep our body temperature at a normal level. They also protect our brains. So when we lose water through our breath, sweat, feces, and urine, it needs to be replaced. If we don't do so we can become dehydrated. That's not a good state of affairs.

The best beverage choice is water. It quenches our thirst better than just about anything. It's calorie, fat, and sugar free. You can't go wrong with no calories. When we choose water over high-sugar beverages, we can decrease our sugar and calorie consumption. This may then reduce our risk for obesity and type 2 diabetes.

By the time you realize you're thirsty, you're already a bit dehydrated. Here are some indicators that you may not be consuming enough water:

- *You're often hungry. Thirst can mask itself as hunger.*
- *You're constipated. Along with exercise and fiber, water is part of the triumvirate to help relieve constipation.*
- *You have dark urine. The ideal color of our urine is lacking in color or very pale yellow.*
- *You don't pee much. The average adult should produce about six cups of urine every day.*

- *You feel tired and fatigued. This can be an early symptom of dehydration.*

Complications from dehydration include:

- **Mild heat cramps, heat exhaustion, and heatstroke (potentially life threatening)**—*Can occur if you don't get enough fluids when exercising and sweating profusely.*

- **Seizures**—*This can occur when your electrolytes, like sodium and potassium, get out of whack.*

- **Cerebral edema (swelling of the brain)**—*Can occur when rehydrating with fluids after experiencing dehydration.*

- ***Kidney Failure***—*At this point your kidneys can no longer remove excess fluid and waste from your body. This can be life threatening.*

- **Hypovolemic Shock**—*This is when you experience low blood volume, which leads to a decrease in your blood pressure and less oxygen in the body. This can also be life threatening.*

- **Coma**—*This can occur with severe dehydration that isn't treated quickly and correctly.*

- ***Death***—*The worst-case scenario.*

The Centers for Disease Control and Prevention

reports that 43 percent of people in the United States have less than four cups of water a day. It also found that one in four children don't drink water at all. According to CDC epidemiologist and lead author of the study, Alyson Goodman, MD, the data "likely indicates that many people either choose less healthy beverages to satisfy their thirst or drink little water daily."

In September 2013, First Lady Michelle Obama announced her campaign to get Americans to "drink up" more water. Poland Spring, Evian, Dasani, Voss, Brita, and other companies participated and put the Drink Up logo on their bottles. Houston, Chicago, Los Angeles-county, and Watertown, Wisconsin also joined in the effort.

If you don't get too excited about drinking a glass of tap or bottled still water, here are some ideas to dress things up:

- *Go carbonated. It's my favorite. From plain to flavored, it's delicious.*
- *Add in a bit of fruit like blueberries or pineapple.*
- *Put in some cucumber slices.*
- *Turn the water into tea (herb or decaf are the better choices). Again, my go-to.*
- *Squeeze a lime, lemon, or orange in the glass.*
- *Pour zero-calorie syrup over crushed ice.*

Our fluid needs depend on several factors, including where we live, our physical activity levels, and our health status. So how do we determine our water needs? One method is the replacement approach. It takes into account that adults pee out about 6.3 cups of urine a day on average and lose almost four more cups through feces, breath, and sweat. And food comprises approximately 20 percent of daily fluid intake. Given that, drinking eight cups of fluids a day in addition to food should replenish all that's lost. But speak with your health care provider for any questions you have about your specific needs.

While water is the best choice, we can satisfy our fluid needs through other things. Food and beverages like tea, coffee, milk, and more can help make up our fluid intake. Other sources include:

Water

Tea

Coffee

Fruit juice

Vegetable juice

Sports drinks

Carbonated soft drinks

Noncarbonated, sweetened fruit-flavored beverages

Milk

Milk substitutes

Alcohol

Soups

Liquid nutritional supplements

Fruit-flavored gelatin

Ice cream

Popsicles

Ice cubes

So what are you drinking? In the above list, some choices are certainly better than others. Water, tea, and coffee (limit caffeine and don't go crazy on the milk, cream, sugar, etc.), milk and milk substitutes, soups (low sodium, not creamy) and gelatin (sugar free) are good choices. Liquid nutritional supplements are good for people who have decreased appetite and aren't able to get adequate daily calories. Carbonated soft drinks that are caffeine and sugar free are okay in moderation. For many of us, that's true of alcohol as well. Of course, alcohol has calories and if we mix it with a sugary substance, the calories can go through the roof. And alcohol lowers our inhibitions, which can cause us to eat more or differently than we normally would. It also dehydrates us.

What are the not so good choices on the list? Full fat and 2 percent versions of milk and milk substitutes, sports drinks, noncarbonated, sweetened fruit-flavored beverages (unless sugar free), and fruit juice just don't make the grade. They're high in calories and sugar.

Some diseases dictate that we limit our fluid intake. For example, this can be true for people with advanced kidney disease. Please consult your health care provider if you have any questions about it.

What's Your Number?

Again, zero is a good number to aim for in our beverages. But I tell clients to include nonfat or low-fat milk in their diets. Low-sodium, low-calorie vegetable juice and other low calorie drinks are a good choice. But so many of us throw caution, and our waistlines, to the wind with our beverage choices.

Let's take a look at some beverages and their calorie counts:

8 ounces (1 cup) of orange juice: 110 calories
8 ounces of fruit punch: 120 calories
8 ounces of vegetable juice: 50 calories
44 ounces of regular soda: 520 calories
24-ounce energy drink: 330 calories
12-ounce can of regular soda: 150 calories
12-ounce can of diet soda: 0 calories
8 ounces of chocolate milk: 150 calories
32-ounce chocolate shake: 1,160 calories
8 ounces of whole fat milk: 150 calories
8 ounces of 2% milk: 120 calories
8 ounces of 1% milk: 105 calories
8 ounces of fat free/skim milk: 90 calories
20-ounce sport drink: 125 calories
20-ounce café mocha: 490 calories
12-ounce black coffee: 5 calories
5 ounces of wine: On average 120 calories
1.5 ounces of hard liquor: On average 100 calories

12-ounce regular beer: Slightly more than 150 calories
12-ounce light beer: About 100 calories
Tea (black) of any size: 0 calories
Water: 0 calories

Keep in mind that we can take beverages that have no calories or are low in calorie like coffee, tea and water and make them caloric. Adding cream, sugar, honey, etc., to coffee and tea can boost the calories. If you buy a twenty-ounce bottle of SoBe Green Tea and drink the whole thing, you'll get 240 calories. Even water can be too high calorie. For example, a twenty-ounce bottle of Snapple Agave Melon Antioxidant Water has 150 calories. Wow.

Drinking too many high-sugar and/or high-caffeine drinks cannot only affect waistlines, but can be harmful to our health. In 2010, thirty-one-year-old Natasha Harris from New Zealand had a heart attack and died. The Associated Press reported that she drank over two gallons of Coca-Cola every day. This is equivalent to about two pounds of sugar and 970 milligrams of caffeine. Way too much. Apparently she also didn't eat much food and smoked about a pack and a half of cigarettes every day. Also not good. When noting her cause of death, coroner David Crerar said, "Were it not for the consumption of very large quantities of Coke by Natasha Harris…it is unlikely that she would have died when she died and how she died."

She isn't the only one whose soda consumption contributed to cause of death. Paul Inman, a thirty-year-old from the United Kingdom, drank so much Coke (about three liters a day) that his lungs swelled to over four times their natural weight. In fact, it killed him while he was sleeping. A sufferer of Asperger's syndrome, a mild form of autism, he engaged in other excessive behaviors, including at times smoking as much as a pack of cigarettes in an hour.

There can be less extreme ramifications of overdoing it on soda. There's the case of Aussie William Kennewell, who had to get a full set of dentures when he was twenty-five years old. Why? His eight-liter-a-day cola consumption caused him to lose all of his teeth. As if that weren't enough, he also suffered blood poisoning from drinking too much soda.

I'm sure none of you is surprised that drinking excessive amounts of sugary soda can cause a host of health problems, including death. But we can also overdo it on healthier beverages like water. Take the case of forty-four-year-old Briton Andrew Thornton, who for several days drank over seventeen pints of cold water in about eight hours. He did this to stop the pain he was feeling in his gums. This excessive amount of fluid caused his brain to swell. He collapsed at his mother's home and was taken to the hospital, where he died from a heart attack the next day.

In 1974, Basil Brown drank copious amounts of carrot juice. He had ten gallons of it every day for ten days. That's way too much vitamin A. In fact, it was about ten thousand times the amount that's recommended for us. He paid for it with his life, dying as a result of the severe liver damage caused by this overindulgence.

Cutting out one can of regular soda, sugary beverage, or juice (about 140 calories) a day can result in a fourteen-pound weight loss in one year. It can also be beneficial to our health. A 2015 study found that sugary drinks cause 184,000 deaths around the world each year.

So what's the best course of action? Choose low to no calorie beverages and drink adequate amounts. Not too much and not too little.

Researchers at Purdue University found that drinking diet soda every day may be associated with weight gain, diabetes, hypertension, and heart disease. The weight gain might occur when people who drink diet soda splurge more on less nutritious foods because they feel they can accommodate the extra calories. Another theory is perhaps the artificial sweeteners in diet drinks impact our bodies' demand for calories, causing us to eat too much.

It's important to note that most studies on artificial sweeteners like saccharin, aspartame, and sucralose are conducted on animals. The data is then projected on to humans. So more studies need to be done.

There are many success stories of people who kick-started their weight-loss programs by doing just one thing: stopping drinking regular soda. At two hundred and sixty-three pounds, Kim Konkel knew she had to lose weight. She started off by just ditching sugary soda for zero calorie sparkling water, determining that this would result in her cutting 700 calories a day. It worked. She lost twelve pounds in one month. This motivated her to start eating healthier and ultimately adding in exercise. She ended up losing ninety-eight pounds. Courtney Dyer followed a similar path, eliminating regular soda from her diet. Like Konkel, she then moved onto healthier eating. This resulted in her losing one hundred and seven pounds.

A study of people fifty to seventy-one years of age found that those who drank more than four sodas a day were 30 percent more likely to develop depression than participants who didn't drink soda at all. Those studied who drank fruit punch had a 38 percent higher risk than people who didn't have sugary drinks. The researchers found that drinkers of lower calorie sodas, fruit punches, and iced teas had a slightly higher depression risk as well.

The guidelines at the hospital where I worked were that beverages, with the exception of milk, should be ten calories or less. This is a good recommendation. I typically get no more than fifty-five calories a day in my beverages. The water and the decaf tea I drink have no calories. I usually have a small can of low sodium V-8 juice every day, which clocks in at thirty calories. And my dessert after dinner? It's a cup of diet hot chocolate that has twenty-five calories.

And full disclosure here, I've been known to indulge in a glass of wine or two from time to time. I certainly enjoy a good party. But we have to be mindful of our intake.

The guidelines for alcohol are no more than one drink a day for females. Males shouldn't have more than two drinks a day. However, remember alcoholic beverages are caloric, particularly the fruity concoctions. So moderation is key. And there are some diseases, such as liver disease and others, and medications, like Metformin and others, that require us to either abstain entirely from alcohol or limit consumption. If you have any questions about your particular case, please ask your health care provider.

A serving size of alcohol is 12 ounces of beer, 1.5 ounces of hard liquor, and 5 ounces of wine. If you have an alcohol dependency, are pregnant, have a condition, or are taking medication that's exacerbated by alcohol, please abstain. I don't recommend drinking alcohol by itself. If you have a drink, I would do so with a meal.

What's the takeaway here? From alcohol to juice and

beyond, some beverages add to our daily calorie intake. A good rule of thumb is to not drink your calories. It will go a long way to making weight management easier.

Water Facts

- *Tap water has nutrients that typically are filtered out of bottled water. Most municipal water has added fluoride, which helps prevent cavities.*
- *Bottled water can be pricey. The cost of one bottle of water equals about one thousand gallons of tap water.*
- *Fossil fuels and water are used up in the production and transportation of bottled water.*
- *Bottled water generates about 1.5 million tons of plastic waste each year.*

I love this quote by Kevin R. Stone, MD, orthopedic surgeon and chairman of the Stone Research Foundation, "Drinking water is like washing out your insides. The water will cleanse your system, fill you up, decrease your calorie load, and improve the function of all your tissues."

I couldn't say it better.

TEN

Just the Facts, Ma'am...

"There's no question obesity is a central public health concern that the nutrition facts panel can play a role in. It's obviously not a magic wand, but it can be an informative tool."

—Michael Taylor, FDA deputy commissioner

The nutrition facts label has been placed on cartons, cans, and boxes of food items in the United States since 1992. Do you read them? I hope you do. They provide us with knowledge of the makeup of what we're putting in our mouths. That's a good thing. They can help us make better choices, which then aids in managing our weight and our health.

The current nutrition facts label can be confusing. But it's still important to understand it. So let's do just that.

Every Picture Tells a Story

What's the first thing we should look at when we start to peruse the label? I often ask this question in my classes. About 80 percent of the time I don't get the correct answer. Where's the place to start? At the top. It's the serving size and number of servings the item contains.

The FDA has a great food label example at fda.gov. I find it amusing that the dish in question is mac and cheese. But the less nutritious nature of this concoction helps us see how the numbers matter. Let's review it.

Sample Nutrition Facts for Macaroni & Cheese

(1) Start Here ➡

Nutrition Facts
Serving Size 1 cup (228g)
Servings Per Container 2

(2) Check Calories

Amount Per Serving	
Calories 250	Calories from Fat

(3) Limit these Nutrients

	% Daily Value*
Total Fat 12g	18%
Saturated Fat 3g	15%
Trans Fat 3g	
Cholesterol 30mg	10%
Sodium 470mg	20%
Total Carbohydrate 31g	10%

(4) Get Enough of these Nutrients

Dietary Fiber 0g	0%
Sugars 5g	
Protein 5g	
Vitamin A	4%
Vitamin C	2%
Calcium	20%
Iron	4%

(5) Footnote

* Percent Daily Values are based on a 2,000 calorie diet.
Your Daily Values may be higher or lower depending on
your calorie needs.

	Calories:	2,000	2,500
Total Fat	Less than	65g	80g
Sat Fat	Less than	20g	25g
Cholesterol	Less than	300mg	300mg
Sodium	Less than	2,400mg	2,400mg
Total Carbohydrate		300g	375g
Dietary Fiber		25g	30g

The label is based on one serving size, not the whole package. Take a look at the below section of the label.

The Serving Size

Serving Size 1 cup (228g)
Servings Per Container 2

What's the serving size of our mac and cheese? It's one cup. If you have two cups, how many servings are you having? Two. And if you have those two cups, how many calories are you having? The label will tell us.

Amount Per Serving

Calories 250   Calories from Fat 110

If you say five hundred, you're correct. Let's break it down:

• *One serving size of the macaroni and cheese in the above label is one cup. It's 250 calories.*

• *There are two servings per container.*

- *If we have both servings (two cups), then we won't take in 250 calories, since that's the amount for one serving.*

- *We'll take in 500 calories, which is two servings worth.*

What's a Calorie?

A calorie is defined as "a unit of heat used to indicate the amount of energy that foods will produce in the human body." It's the amount of heat that's needed to increase one kilogram of water by one degree Celsius.

The definition is a bit confusing. I love dictionaries, but why don't we break this down in more usable terms:

- 40 calories is low.

- 100 calories is moderate.

- 400 calories or more is high.

- 1 gram of protein has 4 calories.

- 1 gram of carbohydrate also contains 4 calories.

- 1 gram of fat has 9 calories.

A gram is about the size of a paper clip.

The amount of calories we need depends on factors such as gender, height, weight, age, and physical activity levels. I'll provide you with some equations to determine your specific needs in chapter 12.

Full of Fat

Next on the nutrition facts label is total fat, saturated fat, and trans fat. The National Heart, Lung and Blood Institute recommends a diet with between 25 percent to 35 percent of total calories from fat. I agree and typically tell my clients to aim for about 30 percent to give them a round number. If you have heart disease, you might consider a lower fat intake. Studies have shown that very low-fat diets (10 percent to 15 percent of total daily calories) can be effective in reversing heart disease.

As I discussed earlier, unsaturated fats are the most heart healthy and should make up the bulk of the fat calories that we intake. Only 7 percent or less of total calories should come from saturated fat. Trans-fat consumption should be as minimal as possible. Zero is best.

Here's a good equation to help you to determine how many calories and grams from fat you should have daily. We'll use the example of 1,200 calories and 30 percent of total calories of fat as our target.

Calorie intake	<u>1,200</u>
% of calories from fat	x <u>30%</u>
Calories from fat	<u>360</u>
Calories in one gram of fat	÷ <u>9</u>
Daily grams of total fat	<u>40</u>

In reviewing the total fat for the mac and cheese label, we see below that one serving has twelve grams of fat. Since one gram of fat equals nine calories, this equates to 108 calories (rounded up to 110 calories on the label) from fat. Remember that one serving of the cheesy pasta in question is 250 calories. That makes the percentage of calories from fat 44 percent. That's too much.

Total Fat 12g	**18%**
Saturated Fat 3g	**15%**
Trans Fat 3g	
Cholesterol 30mg	**10%**
Sodium 470mg	**20%**

It's high in saturated fat as well. A good guideline is to limit saturated fat to no more than one gram for every one hundred calories. Less is better. As you can see on the above snippet of the nutrition facts label, there are three grams of saturated fat per serving. That's too high.

And don't get me started on the trans fat. There are three grams' worth, which isn't close to zero, which is the target. Look for the words "partially hydrogenated" on the ingredients list. If they're there, it means there's trans fat in the product. Run away.

A quick and easy way to keep total calories from fat in a healthy range is to look for three grams or less of total fat for every 100 calories. So if the item has 200 calories, aim for six grams or less of total fat. If it has 300 calories, look for nine grams or less of total fat and so on.

Cholesterol Check

As already mentioned, the 2015 Dietary Guidelines Advisory Committee recommended easing the suggested limitation of cholesterol intake. With that, I hope you don't plan on throwing caution to the wind and regularly chowing down on liver, kidney, unlimited egg yolks, and the like. Moderation and healthier choices still matter. And again, I recommend you speak to your health care provider to make sure that you're not one of us who still needs to limit cholesterol.

Cholesterol comes from all animal products. If it has a mommy, a daddy, a face, a tail, a wing, a gill, a face or a foot, it has it. The amount ranges widely, so there are definitely better choices. Let's look at our mac and cheese:

Total Fat 12g	**18%**
Saturated Fat 3g	**15%**
Trans Fat 3g	
Cholesterol 30mg	**10%**
Sodium 470mg	**20%**

One serving size of the cheesy pasta has 30 mg of cholesterol.

It's Salty

So many of us have diets way too high in sodium. This isn't good because sodium can, among other things, cause us to hold water and raise blood pressure. On average, Americans ingest about 3,500 mg of sodium per day. That's above the upper recommended limit of no more than 2,300 mg a day. And for those of us over the age of fifty-one, African Americans, and anyone with certain diseases that require reducing salt intake, limiting daily sodium consumption to 1,500 mg or less a day is advised. Some ways to do this include removing the salt shaker from the table and when cooking, limiting processed foods, cured meats and canned goods (except no salt added). And beware of sodium-laden restaurant foods. Again, talk to your doctor about your individual goals.

Total Fat 12g	**18%**
Saturated Fat 3g	**15%**
Trans Fat 3g	
Cholesterol 30mg	**10%**
Sodium 470mg	**20%**

Where does our mac and cheese weigh in? As you can see in the above label it has 470 mg in one serving. That's too much sodium for only one food item in a meal. If you're aiming for only 1,500 mg per day and eating three meals a day, your sodium intake for the whole meal should be 400 mg to 500 mg.

Counting Carbs

We've covered carbs in earlier chapters. They include grains, cereals, rice, pasta, bread, tortillas, beans, peas, starchy veggies, fruit, dairy (protein and carb), sugar, honey, sweets and more. One serving of total carbohydrates equals fifteen grams. So, if we're aiming for forty-five to sixty grams of total carbohydrates per meal (three to four servings), which is what I do and what I recommend to most of my clients, then if we eat one serving of the mac and cheese, we'll have thirty-one grams of total carbohydrates. That's equivalent to about two servings of carbs. If we eat the whole package, we're inching beyond four servings.

	% Daily Value*
Total Fat 12g	18%
Saturated Fat 3g	15%
Trans Fat 3g	
Cholesterol 30mg	10%
Sodium 470mg	20%
Total Carbohydrate 31g	10%

Friendly Fiber

While some of us have to be on a low-fiber diet, most of us can and should get a good amount of it. Many health care professionals and organizations recommend getting between twenty-one to thirty-eight grams daily. I aim for thirty-plus grams a day. I tell my diabetic clients that this is also a good goal for them, unless due to a condition they're fiber restricted.

Remember, fiber helps lower cholesterol, manage blood sugar, keep us regular, and makes us full so we eat less.

Fiber's our friend. Make it your best bud.

So how does our mac and cheese stack up? Let's take a look at that big donut hole on the nutrition facts label. At zero grams of dietary fiber, this dish isn't going to be helpful in contributing to our daily fiber intake goal.

Dietary Fiber 0g	0%
Vitamin A	4%
Vitamin C	2%
Calcium	20%
Iron	4%

The Other Nutrients

Following fiber on the nutrition facts label are vitamins A and C, as well as calcium and iron. While there are many other nutrients, these are the only ones required to be listed. That's because in the United States most of us don't get enough of these nutrients. And we should, because they're good for our health.

A, the Apple of our Eyes

Vitamin A is good for our eyes, teeth, skin, skeletal and soft tissue, and our mucous membranes. There are two types: preformed vitamin A (found in animal sources like dairy products, poultry, meat, and some fish) and pro-vitamin A (contained in plant-based foods such as fruits and veggies).

Many of you have probably heard of beta-carotene, which is a carotenoid (dark-colored pigment) found in plant-based foods. It can turn into vitamin A in the body. Beta-carotene is an antioxidant that protects our cells from damage from free radicals. We've already talked about free radicals. They aren't good for us as they can put us at risk for some diseases, including cancer. They also contribute to our aging process.

Good sources of beta-carotene include cantaloupe, apricots, pink grapefruit, green leafy veggies, winter squash, sweet potatoes, carrots, and pumpkin. The FDA recommends a daily value (DV) of five thousand international units (IU) from animal and plant foods. A better guideline is the retinol activity equivalent (RAE):

Males age fourteen and older: 900 micrograms (mcg)

Nonpregnant or breastfeeding women age fourteen and older: 700 mcg

C, It's Not Just for Colds

Besides helping ward off the common cold, vitamin C may play a role in preventing cancer, heart disease, cataracts, and other eye degeneration. Good sources include citrus fruits, kiwi, strawberries, cantaloupe, tomatoes, potatoes, red and green peppers, broccoli, brussels sprouts, cabbage, and more. Do you see the theme here? It's fruits and vegetables. The DV for vitamin C is 60 mg for those ages four and older.

Calcium…It's Not Just for Bones

Calcium is good for our bones and teeth. It also helps our muscles, nerves, and hearts operate well. Make sure your calcium products and supplements contain vitamin D, which allows us to absorb calcium into our bones. And while not definitive, some studies have shown that the combination of calcium and vitamin D can be protective against hypertension, diabetes, and cancer.

Recommended Dietary Allowance for Calcium

Males

19–71 years: 1,000 mg

Age 71 and older: 1,200 mg

Females

19–50 years: 1,000 mg

Age 51 and above: 1,200 mg

Some of us shouldn't take calcium supplements. Please ask your health care provider about your specific needs.

Strike While the Iron's Hot

Iron is important for our muscle function and our brains. It contributes to the formation of hemoglobin, which is the main carrier of oxygen in our bodies. As such, it's essential; every inch of our bodies requires oxygen.

Excellent Sources of Iron:

Dried beans

Dried fruits

Eggs (yolks are high in cholesterol)

Iron-fortified cereals

Liver (high in cholesterol and vitamin A)

Lean red meat (beef especially)

Oysters

Poultry (dark meat)

Salmon

Tuna

Whole grains

While iron from fruits, veggies, nuts, peas, and beans isn't as easy for us to absorb, sources (in addition to those listed above) include:

Almonds

Asparagus

Brazil nuts

Broccoli

Collard greens

Dandelion greens

Dried peas

Kidney beans

Lima beans

Soybeans

Spinach

To increase absorption of iron, pair it with a vitamin C-rich food. Mixing fish, poultry or lean meat with, for example, dark leafy greens or strawberries can increase the iron absorption from the veggie sources by as much as three times. Conversely, there are foods that impede absorption of iron. These include pekoe and black teas. Calcium also reduces iron absorption.

Iron Needs

Males

14 to 18 years: 11 mg daily

Age 19 and older: 8 mg daily

Females

19 to 50 years: 18 mg daily

51 and older: 8 mg daily

If you're younger than the above listed ages, if you're pregnant, breastfeeding, or have a condition that requires different iron needs, please consult your health care provider. Don't take an iron supplement unless it's been prescribed by your doctor.

What's in a Percentage?

The percent daily value can be a confusing number. It's not based on one serving or even the whole package. It's based on a 2,000-calorie diet. There are quite a few of us, including myself, who shouldn't be consuming that many calories a day. So if we go by the percent daily value we may be sabotaging ourselves by getting more of what we actually need in a day.

For the most part, I tell people to look more on the left side of the nutrition facts label than the right. That's because that side tells you what's in one serving size, unlike the percent daily value. But if you want to peruse the percent daily value, just know that if it's 5 percent or less, it's low. If it's 20 percent or more, it's high. Let's take a look at the whole nutrition facts label again and review some of the percent daily values.

1: Start Here:

Nutrition Facts
Serving Size 1 cup (228g)
Servings Per Container 2

2: Check Calories:

Amount Per Serving

Calories 250   Calories from Fat 110

3: Limit These Nutrients:

	% Daily Value*
Total Fat 12g	18%
Saturated Fat 3g	15%
Trans Fat 3g	
Cholesterol 30mg	10%
Sodium 470mg	20%
Total Carbohydrate 31g	10%

4: Get Enough of These Nutrients:

Dietary Fiber 0g	0%
Sugars 5g	
Protein 5g	
Vitamin A	4%
Vitamin C	2%
Calcium	20%
Iron	4%

Quick Guide to Percentage of Daily Value:

**5% or less is low
20% or more is high**

As we can see, the percent daily value of 470 mg of sodium per serving is 20 percent. That's considered to be high in sodium. Conversely, at zero grams of dietary fiber the percent daily value is the lowest it can be, a big fat zero. Unlike sodium, which we'd like to be low, that's not we want for fiber.

You might have noticed that trans fat, sugars, and protein don't have a percent daily value. In the case of protein, it's not required unless the product is claimed to be high in protein or is for use by infants and kids under four.

We don't see a percent daily value for sugars because there's no recommendation for it at this time. It's recommended to keep calories from added sugars to 10 percent of total daily calories. With regard to trans fat, while we know it's not good for us, no reference value has been established. Again, keep trans fat to zero grams or as close to zero as possible.

It Has What?

Don't forget to take a look at the ingredients list below all the numbers on the nutrition fact label. The first four ingredients listed are the most represented in the product. And a long ingredients list can spell nutrition trouble.

The Wave of the Future

Since around 2003 the FDA has been looking to revise the nutrition facts label in the United States. The items that might be changed include serving sizes. They plan on making them more realistic. Let's face it, that means bigger. For example, a twenty-ounce bottle of soda that's currently listed as 2.5 servings would likely be listed as one serving. I wouldn't exactly call that progress, but in today's world, the reality is that many of us are eating and drinking larger portions.

Other changes that would likely be made include emphasizing calorie content and changing or eliminating calories from fat and the percent daily value. Either way, the information on these labels is great to have. It can help us make better decisions as to what we eat.

In the United States, the FDA allows a 20 percent margin of error on nutrition facts labels and restaurant reporting. I know that's a bit scary. If the label says that one serving has 200 calories, it could actually have up to 240 calories. That's a bummer. So, it's not a perfect system, but it's definitely better than nothing.

Restaurants Get into the Act

By the end of 2016, all restaurants in the United States with twenty or more locations must provide diners nutrition information such as calories, saturated fat, sodium, and carbohydrates. While the information isn't presented in label form, the numbers still mean the same. It's important to read the nutrition menus carefully. For example, sometimes the fine print might say that the info is only for the entrée, not the sides.

But the saying "you can lead a horse to water, but you cannot make him drink," is in play here. Not everyone pays attention to the information provided to them whether on packaged foods or at restaurants. According to Gallup's 2013 Consumption Habits survey on how Americans review, or don't review, nutrition information on packages and in restaurants, only 18 percent looked at restaurant menus and postings and only 32 percent looked at food packaging a great deal of the time. Twenty-nine percent didn't look at restaurants or menu postings at all. And 14 percent never looked at the nutrition info on food packaging.

My husband is one who rarely, if ever, reviews nutrition facts labels and information on packaged foods or at restaurants. He prefers to be kept in the dark. You may agree with that or know someone who does. I understand that it can be disappointing sometimes to actually find out how many calories, fat, carbs, etc., that a dish you want to order may contain. But putting blinders on isn't a good idea. To manage our weight and health, we need to know. So brace yourself and start taking advantage of the provided nutrition information. Your body will thank you.

ELEVEN

Meal Time

"Healthy eating is not about strict dietary limitations, staying unrealistically thin, or depriving yourself of the foods you love."

—Lawrence Robinson, Maya W. Paul, MA, and Jeanne Segal, PhD, of HELPGUIDE.org

Where and when we eat differs vastly among us. Some of us love to cook. Others not so much. Some like fine dining, while there are many of us who prefer less grand fare. Prepackaged and frozen foods, or home delivered ones are the go-to for others. Some of us do a combination of everything. Regardless of where and how we eat, it's important to monitor the type and quantity of the food that we consume.

What's on the Menu

I eat out a lot. Three to four nights a week and lunches out on the weekends is indeed my cup of tea. But from fast food to fine dining, we sure can blow our diets at these establishments. The good news is there's a lot we can do to overcome this.

Just about all restaurants will prepare our food the way we'd like it. I often ask for things to be left off and other things added. For example, it's not uncommon for me to order a salad without the cheese, croutons, bacon, and heavy dressing. I often ask for extra veggies. I always request light dressing on the side, and don't use all of it. On any number of entrées I ask for gravy, butter, cheese, oil, and heavy sauces to be left off the plate.

This dates me, but my friends and family have been known to call me Sally. You know, from the film *When Harry Met Sally*. They do this because of the way I order my food, not the scene with that great line, "I'll have what she's having…"

Are you sometimes at a loss for making healthier choices at restaurants? Here are some tips:

Appetizer: *Shrimp/crab cocktail (shrimp high in cholesterol), grilled artichoke (no butter or aioli), other grilled vegetables (sans butter and oil), fruit, steamed clams (no butter), oysters on the half-shell, sliced tomatoes*

Bread: *Small roll, French bread, breadstick, corn bread, crackers, etc. (One piece of bread is enough. Limit or avoid the butter, oil, honey, jelly, etc.)*

Salad: *Any salad with lots of nonstarchy veggies, spinach or tossed green salad, tomato, onion, cucumber salad, tomato, and cottage cheese or fruit. (For all salads order light dressing on the side.)*

Soup: *Tomato soup (not cream based), vegetable soup, gazpacho, chicken or beef bouillon. (Many soups can be high in sodium content, so read the menu nutrition facts.)*

Fish and Shellfish: *Baked or broiled fish (not breaded), steamed or broiled shellfish.*

Poultry: *Broiled or baked chicken, roast turkey, or turkey burger patty. (Poultry skin should be removed, not eaten.)*

Meat: *Beef kebab (with veggies), broiled sirloin steak, or baked or broiled lamb, and pork chops. (Remove all visible fat.)*

Sides: *Steamed vegetables, plain baked or boiled potato, plain rice or pasta, vinegar-based coleslaw, and salad greens.*

Dessert: *Fruit, sherbet or sorbet, and angel food cake.*

Other dining-out tips include:

- *Order an appetizer as your main entrée.*
- *Split an entrée with someone, or cut it in half and take it home for another meal. (It's a good idea to order the "doggie bag" at the beginning of the meal and put half away before eating. Food that's out of sight is typically kept out of the mouth.)*

Many restaurant entrées and a la carte items are very high in calories. It may surprise you to know that if you ate all of the Bistro Shrimp Pasta at Cheesecake Factory, the calorie content would be the same as if you had five platefuls of fish, brown rice, and veggies. And if you enjoy the two entrée meal with Orange Chicken at Panda Express, it would be equivalent to you eating a turkey sandwich, a salad, three bananas, three apples, and three cups of blueberries. If you're not that hungry and just choose to have a blueberry scone from Starbucks, you would be eating the calorie equivalent of five and a half cups of blueberries.

- *Be wary of all-you-can-eat buffets and unlimited or bottomless refills of fries, pasta, and the like.*
- *Substitute unhealthy sides with more nutritious ones.*

High-fat and high-calorie items include those that are fried, deep fried, crispy, breaded, battered, au gratin, buttered, smothered, with gravy, scalloped, Alfredo, cheesy, and so forth.

So if you get a baked potato that's swimming in butter, you've added a lot of calories and fat. If you add sour cream and cheese, you're piling more fat and calories on.

- *Order salad dressing on the side. Use sparingly.*
- *Limit alcohol.*
- *Avoid sugary sodas, juices, and other high-calorie concoctions. Ask for low-fat or nonfat milk.*
- *Limit or avoid the bread and chip basket. I know it can be delectable, but we can eat more calories from the middle of the table than we need in a whole day.*

Keeping your hand away from the bread or chip basket is a good idea. I know it can be yummy, and for many of us, including me, it can be hard to resist. But it can be a high calorie and fat trap, and when the basket is emptied, what does the server do? He or she brings us more.

If I don't like the bread at a particular restaurant, I decline the basket. And when I like it, I often ask them to skip the basket and just bring me one roll. And I tell them not to bring me another, no matter how much I beg.

If you do enjoy a piece of bread or a roll, don't dredge it in olive oil until it's so saturated that rivers of oil drip off the bread when you lift it to your mouth. That's what my husband does. Really.

- *Order from the light or healthy menu. Many restaurants have them.*
- *Review the nutrition information in the restaurant menu and on the menu boards. They're a great guide.*

- *Go online and review nutrition information on restaurant websites and other websites such as calorielab.com, fatsecret.com, and myfitnesspal.com.*

Kiss the Cook

Cooking at home gives us the most control over how our food is prepared. Eating most, if not all, of our meals at home would be great. But this only works well if we choose nutritious foods, prepare them in a healthy manner, and monitor portion sizes and calorie intake.

A recent British study looked at five hundred and one women twenty to twenty-five years of age who watched cooking shows. The researchers found that those who cooked more often had higher BMIs. It's likely that the recipes used on the shows were high in calories and fat.

Whether we cook a lot, a little, or not at all, we still keep some amount of food and drink in our homes. It's important that we stock our fridges, freezers, and pantries with healthy, nutritious food and beverages. I don't know about you, but if candy, donuts, and other treats find their way into my home, I'll eventually eat them, even if I've asked my husband to hide them and not divulge their whereabouts. I invariably hunt them out and find them. Or I badger my hubby until he delivers the goodies. The best way to avoid this happening is:

- *Don't go grocery shopping when you're hungry. Things can go awry when we do. The times I've done it, I've ended up putting an empty wrapper on the conveyor belt at the checkout counter because I've already eaten the contents.*

- *Make a shopping list and stick to it.*

- *If your grocery store delivers, you might give that a try. Order from your list and you're set to go.*

- *Some people say to only shop the perimeter of the grocery store. That means you're perusing the fruits, vegetables, dairy, meats, poultry, and fish aisles. But I say we also need visit some of the interior aisles. Whole-grain breads, rice, pasta, high fiber cereals, healthy oils like olive, canola and peanut, nuts, and more are typically located somewhere in the middle. But there are also temptations in these aisles. Be strong.*

- *Read the nutrition facts labels on the packaged products before putting them in your basket. If you don't like what you see, shelve it.*

Smart Shopping Tips

Instead of whole milk or 2 percent milk: *Buy nonfat or 1 percent milk, or low-fat soy milk.*

In place of high-sugar beverages like soda, sports drinks, and lemonade: *Get flavored or plain sparkling mineral water, sugar-free flavored water, unsweetened or diet tea, light lemonade, or water with fresh squeezed lemon or lime.*

In place of full-sodium canned vegetables and soups: *Purchase no salt added versions. Flavor with herbs and spices.*

Instead of snack foods like chips: *Buy unsalted nuts, trail mix, yogurt, vegetables like celery, baby carrots, cauliflower, and cherry tomatoes (add a dip like salsa or hummus), popcorn, and pretzels.*

In place of whole milk ice cream: *Try light ice cream, low-fat frozen yogurt, sugar-free frozen fruit bars, sugar-free frozen chocolate bars, sorbet or sherbet.*

Instead of cakes, cookies, pies and other sweets: *Buy sugar-free pudding or Jell-O, graham crackers, angel food cake, and fruit (fresh or try freezing grapes or other fruit for a different type of treat. Also try baked apples with cinnamon or a fruit parfait).*

Instead of high-sugar cereals (over 10 grams of sugar per serving): *Purchase oatmeal, Kashi Go Lean, Shredded Wheat, Wheat Chex, Total, Cheerios, Fiber One Original, or other similar cereals. Aim for at least 5 grams of fiber per serving of cereal.*

In place of white bread and white flour tortillas: *Get whole grain bread or whole wheat or corn tortillas. Look for the words "100 percent whole wheat" or "100 percent whole grain."*

Instead of refined pasta and rice: *Try whole wheat pasta or brown rice.*

In place of mayonnaise: *Get light mayonnaise, plain, low-fat or nonfat yogurt, or mustard.*

In place of whole milk cheese: *Buy low-fat or nonfat cheese.*

Instead of regular salad dressing: *Purchase reduced fat or nonfat salad dressing, vinegar (such as Balsamic), salsa, or lemon juice.*

Sometimes choosing ingredients for recipes can be challenging. I always look to lighten up recipes, whether 1) they've been in the family forever, 2) they're my own creative concoctions or 3) I'm preparing food from cookbooks and magazine recipes, even low-fat and low-calorie ones. In addition to the above shopping tips substitutions, try these:

Instead of:

- *Heavy cream, substitute evaporated skim milk.*

- *Sour cream, use plain nonfat or soy yogurt, light silken tofu, blended low-fat cottage cheese, nonfat sour cream or nonfat buttermilk.*

- *One cup of butter or shortening, try one cup of plain or nonfat yogurt, one cup of unsweetened fruit puree, 2/3 cup of olive oil or canola oil or 2/3 cup trans-fat-free margarine.*

- *One whole egg, try 1/4 cup of egg substitute or 2 egg whites.*

- *Ground chuck, use ground turkey.*

- *Whole milk cheese, substitute nonfat and low-fat cheese.*

I enjoy cooking. I can be creative and make up my own recipes, but I often try recipes from cookbooks and magazines. A favorite of mine is *Cooking Light* magazine. I've been making their recipes for years. And even though they're pretty healthy, I still look for ways to lighten them up further while still keeping the flavor intact.

Snack Time

Think about how many tiny bites of foods that we eat throughout the day. We take little tastes of foods and beverages while cooking, off someone's (hopefully someone you know) plate, and a variety of other ways. Many of us don't think of them when we tally up our daily calories. But they can add up.

Even an extra ten calories a day can cause us to gain one pound in a twelve month period. Here are some examples of ten-calorie bites:

A teaspoon of ketchup

One bite of an orange

One small french fry

One ounce of soda

1/30 of a pastry

1/26 of a burger

1/10 a tablespoon of butter or peanut butter

1/8 a teaspoon of mayo

So we should dial back the wee bites.

Another thing to monitor is the number and calorie content of the snacks we have every day. One to two snacks are plenty. Four, five, six, and more is too much. Remember that snacks are small by definition. They're not meals. I like to keep mine at around one hundred calories or less.

Consuming one hundred more calories than needed every day can result in a weight gain of ten pounds in one year. That's equivalent to perhaps one of your snacks a day. That's an area you might want to take a look at. Make your snacks smart. Here are some ideas:

A piece of fruit (you can also pair this with a piece of low-fat or nonfat cheese, cottage cheese, or a closed handful of nuts)

Nonstarchy vegetables like carrots, broccoli, cauliflower, bell pepper, and tomato (if you want a dip for them try salsa, hummus, or low-fat or nonfat dressing)

3 cups of popcorn (sans butter and salt)

Low-fat crackers with low-fat or nonfat cheese or a small amount of peanut butter

Low-fat or nonfat yogurt

Nonfat or 1 percent milk

Low-fat cottage cheese

Monitoring our portion sizes is one great way to stop weight gain. Balanced meals and appropriate snacks, in size and number, help as well. Moderation wins the race.

Balancing Act

No matter where we eat, we should keep the healthy plate in mind, monitor portion sizes, and not drink our calories. Remember balance is key. Aim for the following daily servings from each food group:

Vegetables: *3 to 5 servings (5 or more is better.)*

Fruit: *2 to 4 servings (If you have high triglycerides don't have more than 3 servings a day. Speak with your health care provider for his or her recommendation.)*

Protein*: 2 to 3 servings (If you have kidney disease, speak with your health care provider about daily recommendations.)*

Bread, rice, pasta, and cereal*: 6 to 8 servings (If you have diabetes, work with your health care provider about recommended carb intake.)*

Milk, Cheese, Yogurt: *2 to 3 servings (If you have kidney disease, speak with your health care provider about daily recommendations.)*

Fats and oils: *3 to 8 servings*

There are other diseases than those mentioned above that may affect what and how much we eat of the different food groups. If you have any questions, speak with your health care provider about your individual needs.

Try to eat less processed, canned, and packaged foods. Focus on fresh veggies, fruits, beans, peas, lentils, whole grains, chicken, fish, and fresh meats.

Out and About

We don't always eat at home or at a restaurant. We find ourselves at other people's houses, theaters and sporting events. On trains, planes, and automobiles. In other states, foreign countries, and more. Sometimes this can be challenging for our healthy diets. So what can we do?

- *Take healthy snacks with you to school, work, meetings, in the car, on planes and trains and while sightseeing. These can include fruit, veggies, nuts, low-fat and nonfat yogurt, pretzels, low-fat and nonfat cheese, popcorn, etc.*
- *Have water on hand.*
- *Stock hotel rooms with healthy snacks and beverages.*
- *Bring low-calorie dishes like salads to parties and dinners at other people's houses.*
- *Bring your own low-fat and nonfat salad dressings to restaurants and more.*
- *Limit alcohol intake.*
- *If you splurge a bit every now and then, don't beat yourself up about it. Parties, vacations, and special occasions should be enjoyed.*

We can typically eat healthy meals at almost every restaurant or venue in which we find ourselves. We can certainly do this at home. It may require you to change a bit. But I recommend giving it a go.

TWELVE

On the Move

"If you're having trouble losing weight or having trouble maintaining weight loss, just get out there and maintain a regular regimen of physical activity. Your risk of mortality is significantly reduced."

—Vaughn Barry, PhD, exercise scientist, Middle Tennessee State University

I often ask my clients who have a dog or a cat what might happen if that pet didn't move that much. Would he or she be at a healthy weight? Likely not. Think of yourself in the same way. If we don't move, we may pay the price.

And exercise can do so much more for us than help us manage our weight. It can also:

- *Maintain the health of our muscles and joints.*
- *Keep our bones healthy and prevent osteoporosis.*
- *Manage blood sugar.*
- *Lower blood pressure.*
- *Improve lipid (cholesterol) levels, including increasing HDL.*
- *Decrease heart disease risk.*
- *Help us sleep better.*
- *Reduce fat and increase lean muscle.*
- *Increase energy levels.*
- *Reduce stress levels, anxiety, and depression.*

I can't think of a more fantastic list.

A ten-minute walk can improve your mood for two hours.

In the weight management classes at a hospital where I worked, we asked the patients if they would take a pill that would do all of the above. Of course most, if not all, of us would. That miracle drug is exercise. But so few of us do it. Why's that? Let's take a look at some reasons and strategies to combat them.

Obstacle

Unmotivated: *Get an exercise buddy.*

Pencil exercise in your calendar as if it's work or another obligation.

Envision your final goal of what you want to achieve.

Remind yourself of what you or others have accomplished by exercising.

Say to yourself you'll just try five minutes and if you still don't want to do it you'll stop. Chances are you won't.

Wear a pedometer and challenge yourself to aim for 10,000 steps a day. That's equivalent to 5 miles.

Think outside the box and choose an activity that you like. All movement is good

No time: *Get up a little earlier. (I know, sometimes easier said than done.)*

Prepare breakfast, pack your briefcase or backpack, lay out your clothes, and do any other morning chores the night before to allow for extra morning exercise time.

Stretch in bed before getting up.

If possible, walk to work, school, shops, etc.

While driving, do butt, thigh, or abdominal contractions. Don't worry, other drivers won't notice.

Break your exercise up into ten-minute sessions.

Exercise at your lunch break.

Don't use the drive-thru. Instead park the car and walk in.

Exercise while watching TV, even if it's something like just marching in place.

Climb stairs, park farther away from entrances, and take the long way around.

Walk your dog.

Play with your kids.

Plan exercise as part of your daily or weekly schedule of things to do.

Too tired: *Don't wait until you're dead on your feet. Choose a time to exercise when you have more energy.*

Try to get more and better-quality sleep.

Begin with just five minutes of exercise. If you're still tired, stop. If not, keep going.

Physical Limitations: *Try chair dancing. There are great DVDs and videos available.*

Choose workouts that you can do such as swimming or other exercises in water.

Try working with a physical therapist or personal instructor who can develop an exercise regimen tailored to you.

Weather: *Have both indoor and outdoor exercise activities in your repertoire.*

If you don't have room for exercise equipment or space to do workout videos, Wii and the like, you can do things like go to the mall and power walk. (Save the shopping for afterward.)

Unsafe area: *Stay out of unsafe areas.*

Exercise with a buddy or buddies.

Go to the mall, YMCA/YWCA, gym, etc.

Get exercise equipment, videos, etc. for home exercising.

Limited funds: *Choose free activities like walking, running, yoga, stretching, pickup basketball games, kick-the-can, etc.*

Check out free YouTube exercise videos.

Don't like to sweat: *Drink water and stay hydrated.*

Choose a time to exercise when you can shower immediately afterward.

Have a towel handy so you can wipe off the sweat.

There's an interesting recent small Finnish study that looked at exercise among ten sets of twins in their midthirties. Both twins were active and exercised most of their lives. But several years earlier, one twin cut back on exercise to less than twice a week. The other twin continued to exercise at least twice a week.

Test results found that the more active twin had a lower body fat percentage, normal insulin response, and better levels of endurance. The less active twin had decreased endurance and insulin response, had seven more pounds of body fat, and less gray matter. Gray matter processes information, especially in the areas that control motor function and balance. The twin who exercised less also had signs of early metabolic syndrome. Metabolic syndrome is a group of conditions that occur together—high blood sugar, high blood pressure, abnormal blood cholesterol levels, and excess fat around the waist—that increase the risk of diabetes, heart disease, and stroke. This is just one of many examples of how lack of exercise catches up with us.

I recently got an indoor swim-against-the-current pool. I put it in my garage and tricked out the room so it doesn't look like a garage anymore. The man who delivered my pool took one look at it and called it a "mermaid paradise." He got that right. I'm in exercise heaven.

A study by researchers at Middle Tennessee State University found that a person's weight didn't necessarily predict risk of early death. It was the person's fitness level. Study participants who weren't fit had double the risk of dying during the study than those who were fit, regardless of weight. As a *Huffington Post* article read, "thin, unfit people had twice the mortality risk as obese fit people."

But most of the people in the study groups were men so there wasn't a good cross-section analysis. Further studies are needed.

Moving Forward

My sister once asked me, "I just walked thirty minutes on the treadmill. How much more can I eat?" I'm sure you've guessed my answer. She was about to make a very common mistake by eating the calories she burned through her exercise, or maybe even more. I told her she didn't need additional food.

Some of us may overestimate the calories we burn during exercise. Remember we need to cut 500 calories a day in order to lose a pound a week. We can do this through diet and exercise. But if we burn 200 calories through physical activity and add 300 more calories during the day, we aren't going to achieve the outcome we want.

Researchers at the United States National Institutes of Health found that study participants who engaged in moderate exercise for at least two and half hours a week, or vigorously for one and a quarter hours a week, increased their life expectancy by as much as four and half years.

We all burn calories differently. Our weights, gender, exertion levels, etc., all play a part. Below are examples of approximate calories burned during thirty minutes of physical activity.

Activity	140-lb Person	160-lb Person	180-lb Person	200-lb Person	240-lb Person
Aerobics (light)	173	195	220	246	294
Aerobics (intense)	237	256	290	327	400
Cycling (13 MPH)	252	288	324	360	432
Martial Arts	342	390	440	490	582
Racquetball (vigorous)	326	382	419	465	570

Activity	140-lb Person	160-lb Person	180-lb Person	200-lb Person	240-lb Person
Rowing Machine	223	255	289	326	400
Running (8- minute mile)	395	450	503	559	668
Running (12- minute mile)	252	288	324	360	432
Stationary Bike (moderate pace)	221	252	284	315	378
Stationary Bike (vigorous pace)	331	378	425	473	567
Swimming (Australian crawl—slow pace)	247	283	318	354	417
Swimming (Australian Crawl—fast pace)	305	349	393	446	528
Walking (2 mph)	89	101	114	127	153
Walking (3 mph)	129	143	160	180	213
Walking (4 mph)	161	186	210	235	278
Weight Training (circuit)	252	288	324	360	432
Weight Training (free weights)	175	201	225	250	300
Yoga	121	139	156	174	209

So if you weigh 180 pounds and you walk at a rate of three mph for thirty minutes, you'll burn about 160 calories. If this is all of the physical activity you engage in that day and you're looking to cut 500 calories a day for a one-pound weight loss in a week, then you need to cut 340 calories from your food intake.

Let's take a look at a 140- to 150-pound person burning calories from a different angle:

Food or Beverage	To Burn Off the Calories
12-ounce Bottle of Tropicana Orange Juice **170 calories**	10 minutes of running at a rate of 6 mph, or... 14 minutes of bike riding at 14 to 16 mph, or... Intense weight lifting for 23 minutes.
2 Slices of Pizza **600 calories**	60 minutes of swimming, or... 2.5 hours of yoga.
Donut **350 Calories**	35 minutes of swimming, or... 54 minutes of walking, or... 60 minutes of yoga.

Food or Beverage	To Burn Off the Calories
Bagel with Cream Cheese **500 calories**	2 hours and 30 minutes of ballroom dancing.
Large McDonald's Fries **500 Calories**	60 minutes of weight training, or... 60 minutes of running at 12 mph, or... 60 minutes of cycling at 13 mph.
1 Hard-Boiled Egg and 1 Cup of Sugar Snap Peas **125 calories**	30 minutes of walking at 3 mph (20-minute mile), or... 30 minutes of yoga.
16-ounce Chocolate Shake from Jack-in-the-Box **800 calories**	60 minutes of running at 8 mph, or... 60 minutes of martial arts AND 30 minutes of yoga.
1 Container of Fage Total Greek Yogurt with Blueberry **140 calories**	About 30 minutes of walking at 3 mph.

Food or Beverage	To Burn Off the Calories
Rockstar Energy Drink **280 calories**	17 minutes of running at 8 mph, or… 22 minutes of biking at 14 to 16 mph, or… 37 minutes of weightlifting at an intense level.
Starbucks Blueberry Muffin **380 calories**	23 minutes of running at 8 mph, or… 30 minutes of biking at 14 to 16 mph, Or… 51 minutes of intense weightlifting.
10 Pretzels **227 calories**	14 minutes of running at 8 mph, or… 18 minutes of biking at 14 to 16 mph, or… 30 minutes of weightlifting at an intense level.
1 Small Apple **55 calories**	Approximately 11 minutes of walking at 3 mph.

Food or Beverage	To Burn Off the Calories
1 Tablespoon of Oil **120 calories**	30 minutes of raking leaves.
1 Cup Raw Carrots **25 calories**	5 minutes of walking at 3 mph.

As you can see, it takes a lot less to burn off the calories of the more nutritious food items. Which would you rather work off, two cups of strawberries at 100 calories or a Starbucks Blueberry Muffin at 380 calories? The reality is you don't really need to work off those strawberries.

Approximately 50.2 million people in the United States are members of a gym or health club. Many use the calories-burned number provided on exercise machines to keep track of their progress. If you're one of them, take note. The machines surveyed in a 2013 study overestimated calories burned by 20 percent.

The recommended guidelines are for adults to exercise a minimum of thirty minutes five days a week. If you need to lose some weight, sixty minutes most days of the week is suggested. This can be done in ten-minute increments. (Children and adolescents should aim for sixty minutes every day.)

It's important to put at least a bit of effort into your exercise. A good guideline to follow is the "talk/sing test." We want to be able to talk while exercising. But if we can sing, we're not working hard enough.

If you aren't currently exercising and the thought of starting out at thirty minutes, five days a week is overwhelming, don't let this stop you. Just start somewhere. Even if you begin at ten minutes of physical activity one or two days a week, that's great. Any movement is better than no movement. Then just keep increasing the time and number of days each week. You'll get there.

It's Not the Peter Principle

Whether you're just embarking on an exercise program or you've been physically active for some time, keep the FITT principle in mind. For those just starting out, it gives basic guidelines. For those of us who are looking to ramp up our exercise routines or push past a weight-loss plateau, the FITT principle can give us guidance as to where we might increase and what changes we might make.

FITT Principle

F = Frequency: *How many days are you exercising? The goal is to be physically active a minimum of five days a week.*

I = Intensity: *How hard are you working out? Are your exercising at a moderate level (sweating lightly, can talk, but not sing)? If not, you might think about picking up the pace.*

If you're already working at a moderate pace and you're not happy with your progress, you might increase to more vigorous activity on some days. When you're exercising at this level, you can't talk or sing, and are breathing hard and sweating. This typically occurs with such activities as high-impact aerobics, jogging, swimming laps, and biking uphill. This isn't for everybody.

T = Time: *How long are you working out? You want to get a minimum of thirty minutes, which can be done in ten-minute increments. If you've hit a plateau or aren't reaping the benefits you want or expect, you might consider increasing the number of minutes you're exercising. Don't forget to warm up and cool down.*

T=Type: *Aerobic exercise like walking, running, swimming, biking, hiking, and group sports gets your heart rate up. Choose activities that you like so you'll stick with it. Add in a couple of days of strength training and flexibility exercises.*

So if you're exercising now, kudos to you! If you aren't, there's no time like the present (some may need clearance from their doctor first). We benefit so much from physical activity. So why choose a more couch-potato route?

THIRTEEN

Calorie Is King

"I never met a calorie I didn't like."

—Anonymous

Calories count. When we consume too many, more than we need on a consistent basis, we're likely to pay for it. Clothes get tighter as the pounds pack on. Our health may suffer. On the other hand, we can also not put enough calories into our bodies, as so many of the fad diets tend to have us do. This can also put us at risk for health problems.

First of all, how do you know if you're not at a healthy

weight? If you're in the obese range, you likely have a very good idea of your weight status. If you're what some call "pleasantly plump" or "chubby," you may or may not know. The following are a few ways to determine a healthy weight.

What's BMI?

Body mass index (BMI) is a height-to-weight ratio. The BMI ranges are:

Less than 18.5: Underweight

18.5 to 24.9: Healthy Weight

25.0 to 29.9: Overweight

Over 30: Obese

There are tons of BMI calculators online, but if you want to figure it out on your own, here's the equation:

Take your weight in pounds and divide it by your height in inches squared. That number is then multiplied by 703. That's your BMI. Let's take an example of someone who is 5 feet tall and 140 pounds:

140# (weight in #)/3,600 (5 feet in inches squared) =.039

.039 x 703 = 27.4

In this case, this person is considered overweight.

Some of you may be old enough to remember the Special K commercial that asked us the dreaded question about our midsection…"Can you pinch an inch?" Well, there's something to be said about that. Another way to see how we're managing our weight, particularly for heart health, is waist measurement. Men, look to have a waist measurement of forty inches or less. Ladies' waists should be at thirty-five inches or less.

I'm sure many of you have heard of ideal body weight (IBW). A lot of people in the health care field like to use this benchmark. The drawback is that many of us haven't been at our IBW for a long, long time. We may find it difficult to achieve. But it's something you might want to take a look at. Here's the formula:

Females—*Add 100 pounds for the first 5 feet in height. Then give 5 pounds for every inch over that. You can subtract or add 10 percent from that number using the size of your individual body frame as a guide.*

Males—*Add 106 pounds for the first 5 feet in height, then 6 pounds for every inch thereafter. You also can have the +/− 10 percent range based on body frame size.*

Here's an example of IBW for a 6-foot male:

100 (first 5 feet of height) + 72 (5 inches for every inch over 5 feet) = 172

172 +/− 10% = 155 to 189 pounds

Where do you sit with regard to your weight? How do we reach a healthy weight or if we're there, how do we maintain it? We need to consume appropriate calories.

There are several different ways we can determine how many calories we need in a day. A very simple and general method (not necessarily taking into account all physical activity levels) is:

Women

5'4" or less in height—1,200 calories a day

5'5" or greater in height—1,500 calories a day

Men

5'10" or less in height—1,800 calories a day (Maybe less for men of shorter stature.)

5'11" or greater in height—2,000 calories a day

The gold standard of determining calorie needs is the Mifflin-St. Jeor equation. If you want, you can get out your calculator and do the math.

Males

10 x weight (kg) + 6.25 x height (cm) − 5 x age (y) + 5

Females

10 x weight (kg) + 6.25 x height (cm) − 5 x age (y) − 161

Conversion Key:

kg = pounds divided by 2.2
cm = inches x 2.54

The number you get from the above equation is your basal metabolic rate (BMR)—calories needed while at rest. Once you get this number, you need to multiply it by an activity factor as follows:

1.2 = *sedentary (little or no exercise)*

1.375 = *light activity (light exercise/sports 1–3 days a week)*

1.55 = *moderate activity (moderate exercise/sports 3–5 days a week)*

1.725 = *very active (vigorous exercise/sports 6–7 days a week)*

1.9 = *extra active (very vigorous exercise/sports and physical job)*

Once you multiply in the activity factor, you'll get the number of calories needed to maintain your weight. Don't overestimate your exercise level. Many of us do just that and then we overshoot our calorie needs.

In order to lose weight, you need to cut 500 calories a day to lose one pound a week, or 1,000 calories a day to lose two pounds a week from your calculated daily calorie intake. This can be done through diet and exercise. Remember, don't go below 1,200 calories a day without medical supervision.

If you've figured out your weight and BMI, and measured your waist only to find out that you're not in a healthy range, don't despair. There's something you can do about it. All you have to do is start. Pick one thing and go.

FOURTEEN

The Times They Are a-Changin'

"Change is a process, not an event."

—Harvard Health Publication

Who likes change? Some of us do and kudos for that. But for many, including myself, change is extremely hard. We go kicking and screaming into it and through it. But that doesn't make it impossible. And the reality is that weight management requires behavior change. There's no way around it. But we have to be ready to take the leap.

By reading to the end of this book, you're likely ready. Or maybe you're a bit on the fence. There are several stages of change. Let's take a look at them.

Stages of Change

There are five stages of change. We may find ourselves rotating through all five of them at one time or another for the same issue. The stages are:

- **Precontemplation:** *At this stage, we aren't necessarily even aware of the problem at hand, or are barely so. Therefore we have no plan to change our behavior.*

- **Contemplation:** *We're at the point where we know that there's a problem and we're thinking about what to do to tackle it. But we haven't made the commitment to act.*

- **Preparation:** *This is when we're getting ready to do something about the problem in about thirty days.*

- **Action:** *Ready, set, go! We're now off and running and making changes.*

- **Maintenance:** *We have to work to maintain our changes and avoid relapse. We want to maintain for six months to help ensure long-lasting change.*

Where do you find yourself in the stages of change? If you're not at action, what will it take for you to get there? We all have different motivations.

Another way to look at it is a confidence level of readiness to change. On a scale of one to ten, we want to be at seven or above. I've been known to be able to inch people up to that seven confidence level in my classes and consults. In the pages ahead, we'll cover behavior change more in depth and I'll give you tips for setting goals and achieving them.

Long-lasting behavior change isn't typically a result of fad dieting. If, for example, we cut out certain foods or entire food groups or rely on food that's delivered or made for us, what have we learned and what sustainable behavior change results?

As you reflect on all the information discussed throughout this book, you may find you have just a few things to work on. Or your list may be a long one. Either way, I don't want you to be overwhelmed. This can result in us doing nothing.

I tell my clients that we don't have to change everything overnight. I've already touched on a lot of things you may want to tweak, including portion control, healthier food picks and engaging in physical activity. Start with a few things and then build on those. Mix simpler ones like reading nutrition fact labels with more challenging ones. Keep it going. Small steps lead to big changes.

Some moves we might need to make are either more emotional or cerebral in nature. The following sections may give you more to think about.

Love Yourself

I have taught a lot of weight management classes. One was a twelve-week series that required the participants to keep food diaries, exercise plans, and weekly weigh-ins. It was a fantastic program. When they stepped on the scale, I always listened to how they responded to the weight that was displayed. Some statements I heard:

"I'm bummed, I didn't lose any weight."

"I can't believe I only lost half a pound."

"Oh no, I gained a pound."

These types of responses are termed "negative self-talk." They can be very discouraging and can derail us. Whenever I hear remarks like this, I suggest rephrasing them. Here's a "positive self-talk" spin on the above statements:

"All right! I didn't gain any weight."

"Awesome! I lost half a pound."

"I splurged a bit this week so, I'm glad I only gained one pound."

Which makes you feel better, the negative or the positive statements? Which ones will keep you more motivated? Positivity always wins out.

Weighing yourself every day can turn out to be a negative motivator for some. But it works well for others. Research has shown that weighing daily can aid in weight loss and help us embrace behaviors that help control our weight. So if daily weighing works for you, go for it.

Remember, though, that our weight can fluctuate several pounds on daily basis. So weighing ourselves only once a week can likely give us a more accurate number. This is what I prefer. Either way, remember it's best to weigh yourself on the same scale, at around the same time of day, in your birthday suit prior to eating.

Hunger Games

We should only eat because we're hungry. So many of us eat for other reasons. Depression, stress, boredom, exhaustion, loneliness, and more can lead us to the fridge, vending machine, pantry, and more. This is termed "emotional eating." Sound familiar?

I'm one of those "if I see it, I'll eat it" girls. During the holidays, we spend a lot of time visiting with my mother-in-law in her kitchen. We sit at the table with the family catching up and having fun. There are always cakes, pies, cookies, and pastries on the island and counters. For many years I sat in a chair facing these delectables. After a couple of hours staring at them, I found myself getting up and working my way toward the treats, where I would choose one or two (or three) to eat. It took me a while, but I finally found a solution. I now sit with my back to the holiday desserts. Out of sight, out of mind.

Your emotional eating triggers may be different than mine. It's important to identify what these are and to make a behavior change to combat the urge to eat. This may take time and practice, so don't fret about it. You'll get there. Here are some strategies to help stop eating for reasons other than hunger:

If you have:

Depression:

Try exercising. Even a 10-minute walk or other type of physical activity will help.

Call or speak with a friend or family member.

Watch a comedy. Laughter is great medicine.

Spend time with your pet.

Try therapy.

Boredom:

Get busy and do something you enjoy.

Loneliness:

Call or speak with a friend or family member.

Join a group.

Volunteer.

	Stay busy.
Fatigue:	*Get moving for at least five minutes.*
	Take a nap.
Anger and Anxiety:	*Work it out with exercise.*
	Try relaxation techniques.
	Watch a comedy.
	Try therapy.

Other helpful tips include:

- *Imagining how you'll feel if you don't eat too much.*
- *Finding healthy alternatives for trigger foods that can cause binge eating or raiding of the kitchen.*
- *Keep your kitchen stocked with only healthy foods.*
- *Create a relaxed environment at meal time.*
- *Develop a support system.*

Another way to avoid overeating or making less nutritious choices is to enjoy at least three meals a day. When we skip meals, we may not eat until we find ourselves famished. This can lead to overconsumption.

We should eat when we get the first hints of hunger. We should stop eating when we feel comfortable. Remember, it takes twenty minutes for the stomach to tell the brain it's full. So if we eat until our tummies are stretched to the limit, in less than thirty minutes we'll pay the price. Who's had the feeling your stomach will explode not so long after eating too much food?

It's All in the Mind

Have you ever opened a bag of chips, pretzels, nuts, cookies, candy, or the like and eaten them while on the phone, at the computer or while watching TV? How'd that go for you? Did you eat the whole box or bag and not realize it? Many of us have been there.

A great way to avoid mindless eating is to, well, be mindful of what we're consuming. That means we're paying attention. How do we do that? Here are some tips:

- *Eat sitting down, preferably at a table or counter.*
- *Don't eat in front of the TV, while on the phone, at the computer, etc.*
- *Arrange a nice place setting and lay out the food attractively on your plate.*
- *Enjoy the presentation, color, texture, feel, aroma, and taste of the food.*
- *Put your fork and spoon down frequently. Take your time and savor your food.*

- *If eating with others, engage in conversation.*

On the path to lifelong weight and health management, the majority of us will experience setbacks. That's okay. When you have one, don't beat yourself up about it. Just learn from it and move on. We're human after all.

Goal!

Would you drive from California to New York without a map or travel itinerary? Most of us wouldn't. The same can be said for our weight and health management. We need a plan.

At the beginning of this chapter I talked about taking small steps to achieve big results. This is a manageable way to go. And it's best done through goal setting.

Your long-term goal is the endgame. Examples are "I want to lose twenty-five pounds," and "I want to lower my total cholesterol to less than two hundred." You need to come up with short-term goals to achieve the final result you're looking for.

When setting short-term goals, it's important to be very specific. You want to answer the questions what, when, where, and how. Just saying something like "I want to exercise more" won't cut it. What does that mean? It's too vague to hold you accountable. A more specific statement would be:

- *"I'm going to exercise on the treadmill for sixty minutes on Monday, Tuesday, Wednesday, Friday, and Saturday mornings."*

Other examples of goal statements include:

- *"I'm going to switch from whole milk to 1-percent milk."*
- *"I'm going to sit at the kitchen table for every meal that I eat at home."*
- *"I will make a shopping list and stick to it every time I go to the grocery store."*

As you can see, the above short-term goals aren't ambiguous. We can hang our hat on them. You also don't see the word *try*. It's essential we have a strong confidence level so we can meet the goals we set for ourselves. If we set one that's too far out of reach, we might be sabotaging our efforts. Stretch yourself a bit, but keep your expectations reasonable.

An excellent weight management tool to help us reach our goals is keeping a food and exercise diary. Studies show that people who do this tend to lose more weight and keep it off.

Are the wheels turning in your mind? Are you ready to set some goals? There's no time like the present.

LISA TILLINGER JOHANSEN

FIFTEEN
Mixing It Together

"Choose a change that you can make today, and move toward a healthier you."

—Healthy Eating Tips from choosemyplate.gov

We've covered a lot of information over the last fourteen chapters. How are you feeling? I hope you're not overwhelmed. Remember you don't have to change everything overnight. Just pick a couple of things and start with those. Then build on them with a few more changes each week. Here are some starters. Pick a few and keep adding in more.

- *Eat three meals a day (or smaller, more frequent meals).*
- *Don't skip meals.*
- *Aim for balance by following the healthy plate guidelines. One-half of the plate is nonstarchy veggies, one-quarter of the plate is starch, and the other quarter is lean protein. Fruit and low-fat or nonfat dairy are outside of the plate.*
- *Monitor portion size.*
- *Make at least half of your grains the whole grain variety.*
- *Eat more fruits and veggies.*
- *Limit concentrated sweets and high-fat foods.*
- *Prepare food in a healthy manner, including baking, broiling, steaming, and roasting.*
- *Don't take something healthy and make it less so by loading it up with butter, gravies, sauces, cheese, and the like.*
- *Don't drink your calories. Drink water, low-calorie beverages like tea and coffee, and 1 percent or nonfat milk. Limit or avoid juice and other sugary and high-calorie drinks.*
- *Limit sodium intake. Guidelines are less than 2,300 mg a day unless you're fifty-one years-of-age or older, African American, or have a condition that requires a further cut back on sodium consumption. Then aim for 1,500 mg a day, or less if your doctor recommends it.*
- *Cut back on added sugars.*
- *Aim for twenty-one to thirty-eight grams of fiber a day, unless you're fiber restricted.*
- *Read nutrition facts labels on packaged items and nutrition menus at restaurants.*
- *Eat slowly. Again, it takes twenty minutes for the stomach to tell the brain it's full.*

- *Use a smaller plate.*
- *Plate your food in the kitchen. Don't set bowls of food on the table.*
- *Eat sitting down.*
- *Practice mindful eating. Be aware of the food you're eating. Enjoy it.*
- *Don't eat while watching TV, talking on the phone, while at your computer, etc.*
- *Keep a food diary. This helps you determine what and how much you're eating.*
- *Eat only for hunger. And don't wait until you're starving to eat. You'll likely overeat.*
- *Stop eating when you're comfortable, not when you're full.*
- *Exercise a minimum of thirty minutes most days of the week. Sixty minutes most days of the week is better for weight loss.*
- *Wear a pedometer and aim for ten thousand steps (five miles) a day.*
- *Get adequate sleep.*
- *Employ positive self-talk.*
- *Don't beat yourself up if you deviate from healthy eating. Learn from it and move on.*
- *Take advantage of your support system. This can be a friend, family member, group, or more.*
- *Set short-term goals to help you reach your long-term ones. Be very specific and hold yourself accountable.*
- *Eat appropriate calories.*
- *Remember, slow and steady wins the race.*

I Get By with a Little Help from My Friends

For a lot of us, a bit of guidance and support is a huge help in our efforts to be healthy. We've already talked about the reversal diet, the DASH diet, and the Mediterranean diet. Any of these would be a good choice for your eating plan for life. Check out appendix A of this book for websites that will give you more information on them. Let's take a look at some other plans that you might find helpful.

Weight Watching

Many health care professionals, including me, like Weight Watchers and I've recommended it to a lot of people. The program assigns points to foods, with the lowest points going to healthier, more nutritious choices. Fruits and nonstarchy vegetables are unlimited. Each member gets an assigned number of points based on individual goals and spends those points throughout the day through appropriate, balanced meals and snacks. Daily calorie intake doesn't dip below 1,200.

Weight Watchers provides online and in-person support. This is great for those who need it. Overall it's a good plan. My only caveat is that it isn't disease specific. For example, someone with diabetes or high triglycerides shouldn't be having unlimited fruit. We need to marry our own personal dietary needs into our diet plans.

It Speaks Volumes

While it may require a bit more thinking than I like, Volumetrics offers a sensible weight-loss approach. This diet is based on feeling full, not deprived. The focus is to fill up on healthier and lower-energy dense foods that have fewer calories, but more volume. By doing this you can eat more, but take in fewer calories. Exercise also plays an integral role.

There are four categories of food on this plan:

Category 1: *Broth-based soups, fruits, nonstarchy vegetables (like broccoli, green leafies, bell peppers, and more). These foods are considered free. You can enjoy them anytime.*

Category 2: *Whole grains, legumes, lean protein, and low-fat dairy in proper portion sizes.*

Category 3: *Cheese, high-fat protein, bread, fat-free baked snack goods, and desserts. Only small servings of these are advised.*

Category 4: *Nuts, fats, fried food, cookies, and candy. I'm sure you guessed it: these are not a go-to and should be "sparing" in portion size.*

The diet's focus is on foods that contain a lot of water and fewer calories. A follower must be aware of energy-dense foods. These are foods that have a lot of calories in small amounts. Writing for WebMD, dietitian Kathleen M. Zelman had a great example of this. It compared the calories in a big bowl of soup to the energy-dense cheeseburger. You could either eat the entire bowl of soup or one-sixth of the burger. That's a no-brainer.

This diet may require more thinking than some of us would like, and I don't consider nuts to be in the same category as desserts and fried food. But if you're up for it, give it a try.

Bring Home the Bok Choy, Sauté It Up in the Pan

Earlier I mentioned *Cooking Light* magazine. If you like to cook but need help in menu planning and a bit of support, you might try the *Cooking Light* diet. You input your preferences online, and each week you're e-mailed all the recipes you need for the next seven days. Don't worry, they allow for nights out. It costs, so be aware. I like the recipes, but if you don't need a set weekly meal plan, you could also just peruse the magazine or their website for recipes to try.

It's Not Over, It's Just Beginning!

Congratulations! You've reached the end of the book. I hope you've found it helpful and you're ready to chart your healthy course. If you have any questions, I'm happy to answer them. Please check out the Q&As on my website or contact me at consultthedietitian.com. You can also visit my Facebook page at Lisa Tillinger Johansen, follow me on Twitter at Lisa T. Johansen, and visit my other websites stopthediet.com and fastfoodvindication.com. In addition, please check out appendix A, where I've listed a host of other websites and resources you might find helpful.

Good luck. I know you can do it!

LISA TILLINGER JOHANSEN

APPENDIX

In addition to my websites **consultthedietitian.com, stopthediet.com** and **fastfoodvindication.com,** here are some other websites that I recommend:

Academy of Nutrition and Dietetics – eatright.org

Ask the Dietitian – askthedietitan.com

American Diabetes Association – diabetes.org

American Heart Association – heart.org

Asthma and Allergy Foundation of America – aafa.org

Calorie King – calorieking.com

Centers for Disease Control and Prevention – cdc.gov

Celiac Disease Foundation – celiac.org

Cooking Light – cookinglight.com

Dairy Council of California (healthy eating made easier) – mealsmatter.org

DaVita (kidney disease and dialysis information) – davita.com

Eating Well – eatingwell.com

Everyday Health (health information, resources, tools and news) – everydayhealth.com

FitDay (free weight loss and diet journal) – fitday.com

Food Addicts Anonymous – foodaddictsanonymous.org

Food FIT (healthy low fat recipes, diet plans, holiday recipes and free online diets) – foodfit.com

Food Safety (federal food safety information) – foodsafety.gov

LIVESTRONG (lose weight and get fit with diet, nutrition & fitness tools) – livestrong.com

Mayo Clinic – mayoclinic.com

My Fitness Pal (free calorie counter, diet and exercise journal) – myfitnesspal.com

National Institutes of Health – nih.gov

Ornish Lifestyle Medicine – ornishspectrum.com

Overeaters Anonymous – oa.org

SparkPeople (free diet plans, food and fitness trackers and more) – sparkpeople.com

The National Kidney Foundation – kidney.org

United States Department of Agriculture (USDA) Choose My Plate – choosemyplate.gov

WebMD – webmd.com

Weight Watchers – weightwatchers.com

REFERENCES

3 Fat Chicks. (n.d.) *The Lindora diet.* Retrieved from
http://www.3fatchicks.com/the-lindora-diet/

ABC Health & Wellbeing. (2013, May 30). *Is eating too much wheat bad for your health?* Retrieved from
http://www.abc.net.au/health/talkinghealth/factbuster/stories/2013/05

ABC News. (2012, January 5). *Chris Powell's tips for eating carbs to drop the pounds.* Retrieved from
http://abcnews.go.com/blogs/health/2012/01/05/chris-powells-tips-for-eating-carbs-to-drop-the-pounds/

ABC News. (2012, May 8). *100 million dieters, $20 billion: Weight-loss industry by the numbers.* Retrieved from http://abcnew.go.com

ABC News. (2014, May 28). *All about yacon: what it is, and what it may do for weight loss.* [Web log post]. Retrieved from
https://gma.yahoo.com/blogs.abc-blogs/yacon-may-weight-loss-134110380-abc-news-heatlh.html

ABC Science News. (2013, February 19). Mesolithic hunter-gatherers had much healthier mouths than modern humans. *Discovery News.* Retrieved from http://news.discovery.com/human/evolution/ancestors-had-much-better-teeth-130219.htm

Access Hollywood. (2013, April 5). *Gwyneth Paltrow sets record straight on her kid's carbs: they love 'hot cheetos & coke'* Retrieved from
http://news.yahoo.com/gwynethpaltrow-sets-record-straight-her-kids-carbs-200231380.html

AceShowbiz. (2012, April 11). *Miley Cyrus' gluten-free diet encouragement met with backlash from experts.* Retrieved from
http://www.aceshowbiz.com/news/view/00049552.html

Agatston, A. & Signorile, J. (2008). *The south beach diet super charged*. New York, NY: Rodale, Inc.

Allen, J.E. (2012, April 5). Raspberry ketones frenzy follows Dr. Oz show. *ABC News*. Retrieved from http://abcnews.go.com/Health/Diet/raspberry-ketones-frenzy/story?id=16074044.

Allrich, K. (n.d.). The g-free diet: an opinion from Elaine Monarch, CDF. [Web log post]. *Gluten-Free Goddess*. Retrieved from http://glutenfreegoddess.blogspot.com/2009/05/g-free-diet-opinion-from-elaine-monarch.html

Almendrala, A. (2013, November 20). Fat but fit? Study reveals that fitness, not weight, predict risk of early death. *The Huffington Post*. Retrieved from http://www.huffingtonpost.com

Almendrala, A. (2015, January 16). What the world's healthiest diets have in common. *The Huffington Post*. Retrieved from http://www.huffingtonpost.com

Alphonse, L.M. (2013, June 10). Corset-wearing German woman's scary 16-inch waist: What are the risks? *Yahoo! Deutschland Lifestyle*. Retrieved from http://de.lifestyle.yahoo.com/

American Diabetes Association & American Dietetic Association. (n.d.) *Choose Your Foods*. Alexandria, VA, Chicago, IL.

American Dietetic Association. (n.d.). *Portion size tips*. Retrieved from www.eatright.org

Amidor, T. (2014, January 24). Top fad diets: love them or leave them? [Web log post].

U.S. News. Retrieved from http://health.usnews.com/health-news/blogs/eat-run//2014/01/24/top-fad-diets-love-them-or-leave-them

Amos, C.L (2008, May). The impact of visceral influences on consumers' evaluation of weight loss advertising. *UNT Digital Library*. Retrieved from http://digital.library.unt.edu/ark:/67531/metadc6138/

Ancestral Weight Loss Registry. (n.d.). *Safety and efficacy of diets low in carbohydrates*. Retrieved from http://www.awlr.org/carb-restricted-diets-html

Anderson, J. (2011, October 23). Celiac disease & gluten sensitivity. *About.com*. Retrieved from http://celiacdisease.about.com.od/copingwiththediet/a/Gluten-On-Food-Lables.htm

Anderson, J.C. (2011, November 8). Weight Watchers works: Study. *The Huffington Post*. Retrieved from http://www.huffingtonpost.com/

Anonymous. (2010, October 28). In 1974, a British health nut drank himself to death with carrot juice. *OMG Facts*. Retrieved from http:www.omg-facts.com/Science/In-1974-A-British-Health-Nut-Drank-Himse/17490

AP. (2011, September 3). New food nutrition labels from FDA coming. *CBS News*. Retrieved from http: gwyneth-paltrow-elimination-diet-new-cook-book-to-help-fans-lose-real-weight//www.cbsnews.com/2100-201_162-20101420.hmtl

Archer, D. (2013, October 7). Reading between the (head) lines. *Psychology Today*. Retrieved from https://www.psychologytoday.com/blog/reading-between-the-headlines

Arciero, R. (2013, March 13). Gwyneth Paltrow elimination diet: new cook book to help fans lose 'real' weight. *Examiner*. Retrieved from gwyneth-paltrow-elimination-diet-new-cook-book-to-help-fans-lose-real-weight

Ask Men. (2013, May 7). *15 snacks you eat at work that tae you way too long to burn off the calories*. Retrieved from http://www.thepostgame.com/blog/list/201305/15-snacks-you-eat-work-take-you-way-too-long-burn#1

Associated Press. (2014, June 18). Dr. Oz grilled in congress, admits weight loss products he Touts don't pass 'scientific muster.' *The Huffington Post*. Retrieved from http://www.huffingtonpost.com/

Associated Press. (2015, January 8). *5 things to look for as government writes new dietary advice*. Retrieved from https://www.yahoo.com/health/5-things-to-look-for-as-government-writes-new-107508680492.html

Avila, J. (2013, January 8). Calorie counts: how accurate are they? *ABC News*. Retrieved from http://abcnews.go.com/Health/calorie-counts-accurate/story?id=18164180

Barnard, N.D. (2011). *21-day weight loss kickstart*. (2011). New York, NY: Grand Central Life & Style.

Batur, J. (2012, December 14). Miley Cyrus, Victoria Beckham, Jessica Alba and more go gluten-free. *E! Online*. Retrieved from http://www.eonline.com/news/371344/miley-cyrus-victoria-beckham-jessica-alba-and-more-go-gluten-free

Bauer, J. (n.d.) The juicing craze: health or hype? *Food Cures*. Retrieved from http://www.joybauer.com/

Bays, J.C. (2009). *Mindful eating*. Boston, MA: Shambhala Publications, Inc.

Be Well. (n.d.). *Resting metabolic rate (RMR)*. Retrieved from http://www.bewelldowell.org/bewell/content.php?page=restingmetabolicrate

Bedwell, S.J. (2015, January 8). The non-diet secret to losing the weight for good in 2015.

SELF. Retrieved from http://www.self.com/flash/health-blog/2015/01/non-diet-secret-losing-weight-good-2015/

Beil, L. (2013). How a fruit juice cleanse affects your body. *Women's Health*. Retrieved from http://www.womenshealthmag.com/weight-loss/detox-diet-side-effects

Belluz, J. (2014, August 25). Dr. Oz's 3 biggest weight loss lies, debunked. *Vox.* Retrieved from http://www.vox.com/2014/8/25/6063521/dr-oz-lies

Belluz, J. (2014, September 20). How to rearrange your environment to lose weight. *Vox.* Retrieved from http://www.vox.com/2014/9/20/6513197/brian-wansink

Belluz, J. (2014, December 17). Scientists tallied up all the advice on Dr. Oz's show. Half of it was baseless or wrong. *Vox.* Retrieved from http://www.vox.com/2014/12/17/7410535/dr-oz-advice

Belluz, J. (2014, December 27). Meet the anti-Dr. Oz: Ben Goldacre. *Vox.* Retrieved from http://www.vox.com/2014/12/27/7423229/ben-goldacre

Belluz, J. (2015, January 26). Government confirms one of Dr. Oz's favored diet pills is a total hoax. *Vox.* Retrieved from http://www.vox.com/2015/1/26/7916745/green-coffee-bean

Belluz, J. (2015, April 16). A group of doctors just asked Columbia to reconsider Dr. Oz's faculty appointment. *Vox.* Retrieved from http://www.vox.com/2015/4/16/8423867/dr-oz-letter-columbia

Belluz, J. (2015, April 20). Dr. Oz launches his counterattack against the doctors questioning his credibility. *Vox.* Retrieved from http://www.vox.com/2015/4/20/8455505/dr-oz-GMO

Belluz, J. (2015, June 13). The American Medical Association is finally taking a stand on quacks like Dr. Oz. *Vox.* Retrieved from http://www.vox.com/2015/6/13/8773695/AMA-dr-oz

Better Health Channel. (n.d.). *Weight loss and fad diets.* Retrieved from http://www.betterhealth.vic.gov.au/bhcv2/bhcarticles.nsf/pages/Weight_loss_and_fad_diets

Bever, L. (January). Urban outfitters told to remove online ad featuring 'too skinny' model. *The Washington Post.* Retrieved from http://www.washingtonpost.com

Blanchard. P. (2013, June 24). Health report: American medical association labels obesity a disease. Retrieved from http://whcuradio.com

Blanck, H.M., Khan, L.K. & Serdula, M.K. (2004, December). *Prescription weight loss pill use among Americans: patterns of pill use and lessons learned from the fen-phen market withdrawal.* Retrieved from http://www.ncbi.nlk.nih.gov/pubmed/15539063

Blanco, M. & Pendleton, J. (2013). *The coconut oil diet.* New York, NY: Alpha Books.

Blanco, M. & Pendleton, J. (2013). *The complete idiot's guide to the coconut oil diet.* New York, NY: Alpha Books.

Blickley, L. (2013, November 26). How Kelly Osbourne dropped 70 pounds, and kept the weight off. *The Huffington Post.* Retrieved from http://www.huffingtonpost.com

Bloom, S. (2013, May 28). Dietitian: overeating an assault on the body. *USA Today.* Retrieved from http://www.usatoday.com/

Boboltz, S. (2014, September 4). This is what people ate in the 18th century. Be happy you're alive today instead. *Huffington Post.* Retrieved from http://www.huffingtonpost.com/

Brainy Quotes. (n.d.). *Robert Atkins quotes.* Retrieved from http://www.brainyquote.com/authors/r/robert_atkins.html

Brandi & Diets in Review. (2013, August 3). Debunking the 5:2 diet. *Care2 Healthy Living.*

Retrieved from http://www.care2.com/greenliving/debunking-the-52-diet.html

Brewer, R. (2013, July 15). Three weight loss companies just got a huge boost. *The Motley Fool.* Retrieved from http://www.fool.com

Brodesser-Akner, T. (2011, August 2). When dieting becomes a role to play. *The New York Times.* Retrieved from http://www.nytimes.com

Brooke, C. (2008, July 8). Man dies of water overdose after drinking 17 pints in eight hours to soothe sore gums. *Mail Online*. Retrieved from http://www.dailymail.co.uk

Brown, A. (2013, August 9). In U.S., less than half look at restaurant nutrition facts. *Gallup*. Retrieved from http://www.gallup.com/poll/163904/less-half-look-restaurant-nutrition-facts.aspx

Brown, J. (2013, July 25) I lost weight: John M. Brown lost 130 pounds with the help of a paleo diet. [Web log post]. *HuffPost Healthy Living*. Retrieved from http://www.huffingtonpost.com/

Byrd, L. (2012, February 14). Fad diets and gimmicks are a fat business. *Michigan State University Extension*. Retrieved from http://msue.anr.msu.edu/news/fad_diets_and_diet_gimmicks_are_a_fat _business.

Callahan, M. (2015, January 18). The brutal secrets behind 'the biggest loser' *New York Post*. Retrieved http://nypost.com/Calorie, Fat and Carbohydrate Counter, 2011 Edition. Costa Mesa, CA: Family HealthPublications.

Calorie Lab. (n.d.). *Cheesecake factory calorie counter*. Retrieved from http://calorielab.com/news/2007/07/28/calorie-pusher-comes-to-town-the-cheesecake-factory-hits-rochester/

Campbell, T.C. & Campbell, II, T.M. (2006). *The china study*. Dallas, TX: BenBella Books, Inc.

Cameron, P. (2009, July 20). What is the Hollywood diet? *LiveStrong*. Retrieved from http://www.livestrong.com/article/17202-hollywood-diet/

Cannady, A.J. (2013, November 26). The dukan diet. *WebMD*. Retrieved from http://www.webmd.com/diet/features/dukan-diet-review

Cancer Prevention Research Center. (n.d.). *Transtheoretical model*. Retrieved from http://www.uri.edu/research/cprc/TTM/StagesOfChange.htm

Cardium Health. (2005). *States of Change*. Retrieved from
http://www.cardiumhealth.com/real_caring/a_readiness.html

Carollo, K. (2012, June 27). Atkins-like diets may increase risk of heart
disease. *ABC News*. Retrieved from http://abcnews.go.com/Health

CDC. (n.d.). *Protein*. Retrieved from
http://www.cdc.gov/nutrition/everyone/basics/protein.html

Celebrity Beauty Magazine. (n.d.). *Dr. Oz reveals a natural ingredient he says
will erase 25 lbs of fat in 1 month used by celebrities*. Retrieved from
http://celebbeautmags.com/losefatquickly.html

Central intelligence Agency. (2012). A spotlight on world obesity rates.
Retrieved from https://www.cia.gov/news-information/featured-story-
archive/2012-featured-story-archive/obesity-according-to-the-world-
factbook.html

Cespedes, A. (2010, March 23). 7-day cabbage soup diet. *LiveStrong*.
Retrieved from http://livestron.com/article/91927-7day-cabbage-soup-
diet/

Chang, K. (2013, February 4). Gluten-free for the gluten sensitive.
Everyday Health. Retrieved from
http://well.blogs.nytimes.com/2013/02/04/gluten-free-whether-you-
need-it-or-not/?_r=0

Chatsko, M. (2013, May 18). 25 belt-busting obesity facts. *The Motley Fool*.
Retrieved from
http://www.fool.com/investing/general/2013/05/18/25-belt-busting-
obesity-facts.aspx

Choose Sensible Portion Sizes. (n.d.). *Choosemyplate.gov*

Christensen, J. & Wilson, J. (2014, June 19). Congressional hearing
investigates Dr. Oz 'miracle' weight loss claims. *CNN*. Retrieved from
http://www.cnn.com/2014/06/17/healthsenate-grills-dr-oz/

CLEAN 21-Day Elimination Diet. (n.d.). Retrieved from

http://www.cleanprogram.com/media/files/clean-program-manual.pdf

Cleveland Clinic. (n.d.). *Fad diets.* Retrieved from http://my.clevelandclinic.org/healthy_living/weight_control/hic_fad_die ts.aspx

CMAJ. (2013). *Intermittent fasting: the science of going without.* Retrieved fromwww.cmaj.ca/lookup/doi/10.1503/cmaj.109-4451

CNBC/Off the Cuff. (n.d.) *Weight Watchers CEO: Forget willpower and do this instead.* [Web Log Post]. Retrieved from http://finance.yahoo.com/blogs/off-the-cuff/weight-watchers-ceo-forget-willpower-instead-203715631.html

Collingwood, J. (n.d.). The psychology of diets. *Psych Central.* Retrieved from http://psychcentral.com/lib/the-psychology-of-diets/0001506

Collis, H. (2013, July 8). American Samoas' battle against obesity as 95 percent of the nation are declared overweight. *Daily Meal.* Retrieved from http://www.dailymail.co.uk/

Conlin, J. (2013, March 1). England develops a voracious appetite for a new diet. *The New York Times.* Retrieved from http://www.nytimes.com

Consumer Health Answers. (2013, November). *Bystrictin reviewed: Does bystrictin work?* Retrieved from http://consumerhealthanswers1.blogspot.com/2013/10/how-is-bystrictin-really-different-from.html

Consumer Reports. (2011, January). *Diet taste-off Jenny Craig edges out rival Nutrisytem.* Retrieved from http://www.consumerreports.org.cro/2012/04-diet-taste-off/index.htm

Consumer Reports. (2013, March). *How accurate are chain calorie counts?* Retrieved from http://www.consumerreports.org/cro/magazine/2013/03/how-accurate-are-chain-restaurant-calorie-counts/index.htm

CookDiet.com (n.d.). *Dr. Siegal's cookie diet official store.* Retrieved from http://www.cookiediet.com/?gelid=CIPHguLNpbgCFYN_QgodfykAJg

Cordain, L. (2012). *The paleo diet.* Retrieved from
http://thepaleodiet.com/the-paleo-diet-premise/

Corleone, J. (2014, August 22). Canada's food guide and calorie counter.
LIVESTRONG. Retrieved from
http://www.livestrong.com/article/284951-canadas-food-guide-and-
calorie-counter/

Cosmopolitan. (n.d.). *The Dukan diet everyone (including Kate Middleton) is
obsessing over.* Retrieved from
http://www.cosmopolitan.com/advice/health/the-dukan-diet-kate-
middleton-weight-loss

Cox, L. (2013, January 11). Anne Hathaway drops 25lb on the Les
Miserables lettuce diet…then breaks her superskinny arm. *Daily Mail.*
Retrieved from http://www.dailymail.co.uk/

Cutting Edge. (n.d.). Homocysteine. *John Wiley & Sons Publishers, Inc.*
Retrieved from
http://www.wiley.com./college/boyer/0470003790/cutting_edge/homo
cysteine/homocysteine.htm

Dalessio, J. (2013, January). Weight-loss myths might be keeping us fat.
Everyday Health. Retrieved from
http://www.everydayhealth.com/weight/weight-loss-myths-might-be-
keeping-us-fat-7743.aspx

D'Adamo, P.J. & Whitney, C. (1996). *Eat right for your type.* New York, NY:
G.P. Putnam's Sons.

D'Adamo, P.J. & Whitney, C. (2001). *Eat right 4 your type.* London:
Century Books Ltd.

Daily Dose. (2015, January 27). U.S. bans ads for green coffee weight-loss
supplements. *Health Central.* Retrieved from
http://www.healthcentral.com/dailydose/cf/2015/01/27/u_s_bans_ads
_for_green_coffee_weight_loss_supplements

Daily Mail Reporter. (2012, March 19). Women have tried 61 diets by the age of 45 in the constant battle to stay slim. *Mail Online*. Retrieved from http://www.dailymail.co.uk

Daily Mail Reporter. (2013, May 26). A quarter of fast food diners underestimate their meals by 500 calories – with teenagers and Subway customers the worst. *Mail Online*. Retrieved from http://www.dailymail.co.uk

Davis, K. (n.d.). The fad-diet and weight-loss obsession: year in review 2012. *Encyclopaedia Britannica*. Retrieved from http://www.britannica.com/EBchecked/topic/1887697/

The-Fad-Diet-and-Weight-Loss-Obsession-Year-In-Review-2012 Davis, L. & Clark, D. (2013, February 21). How accurate are exercise machines? *Good Morning America*. Retrieved from http://gma.yahoo.com/accurate-exercise-machines-191237292-abc-news-health.html

Davis, L. (2013, April 8). 'Overnight diet' promises weight loss while you sleep. [Web Log Post]. *ABC News*. Retrieved from http://abcnews.go.com/blogs/health/2013/04/08/overnight-diet-promises-weight-loss-while-you-sleep/

Davis, W. (2012). *Wheat belly...in 30 minutes*. Berkeley, CA: Garamond Press.

Dawson, A. (2013, September 20). Dieter beware: Weight-loss fads can be bad for your health. *Los Angeles Times*. Retrieved from http://www.latimes.com

Denisko, Y. (2010). Laxatives: Proceed with caution. *Consumer Health Information Corporation*. Retrieved from http://www.consumer-health.com/services/LaxativesProceedwithCaution.php

Denke, M.A. (2001, July 1). Metabolic effects of high-protein, low-carbohydrate diets. *The American Journal of Cardiology* 2001; 88:59-61.

Derrer, D.T. (2004, October 5). The protein power diet. *WebMD*. Retrieved from http://www.webmd.com/diet/protein-power-what-it-is?page=3

Detox Diet. (n.d.). *Diabetes.co.uk*. Retrieved from
http://diabetes.co.uk/diet/detox-diet.html

Diabetes.co.uk. (n.d.). *Low carb high fat diet*. Retrieved from
http://www.diabetes.co.uk/diet/low-carb-high-fat-diet.html

Diabetes.co.uk. (n.d.). *Prediabetes (borderline diabetes)*. Retrieved from
http://www.diabetes.co.uk/pre-diabetes.html

Diet. (n.d.). In *Merriam-Webster's online dictionary*. Retrieved from
http://www.meriam-webster.com/dictionary/diet

Diet.com. (n.d.) *3-day diet*. Retrieved from http://www.diet.com/g/3day-diet

Downs, M. (n.d.). Why do we keep falling for fad diets? *WebMD*.
Retrieved from http://www.webmd.com/diet/features/why-do-we-keep-falling-for-fad-diets

Drummond, J. (2012). *The 5:2 diet*. London, England: Kyle Craig
Publishing.

Duell, M. (2013, May 29). Obsessive man who downed three litres of cola
a day died after drink made his lungs swell to four times the normal
weight. *Daily Mail*. Retrieved from http://www.dailymail.com/

Dukan Diet. (n.d.) *Diabetes.co.uk*. Retrieved from
http://www.diabetes.co.uk/diet/dukan-diet.html

Dukan Diet. (n.d.) *Dukan diet plan*. Retrieved from
http://www.dukandiet.com/low-carb-diet

Dukan, P. (2011). *The dukan diet*. New York, NY: Crown Archetype.

Eat This. (n.d.). 20 worst drinks in America. *Mens Health*. Retrieved from
http://eatthis.menshealth.com/slideshow/print-list/184612

Edmundson, A. (n.d.). Diet shakes: sipping to slimness. *WebMD*.

Retrieved from http://www.webmd.com/diet/features/diet-shakes-sipping-to-slimness

Eggenberger, N. (2012, April 10). Miley Cyrus slammed for gluten-free diet. *US Magazine*. Retrieved from http://www.usmagazine.com/celebrity-body/news/miley-cyrus-slammed-for-gluten-free-diet-2012104

Elkaim, Y. (2014). *The all-day energy diet*. Carlsbad, CA: Hay House, Inc.

Ellen's Good News/The Good News. (n.d.). These elementary school students went vegetarian, and the results are astounding. *Shine*. Retrieved from http://shine.yahoo.com

Elliston, Jr., C.B. (2007), *Prevent and reverse heart disease: the revolutionary, scientifically proven nutrition-based cure*. New York, NY: Avery.

eMedExpert. (2009). *How to raise metabolism*. Retrieved from http://www.emedexpert.com/tips/metabolism-tips.shtml

Epilepsy Foundation. (n.d.). *Ketogenic diet*. Retrieved from http://www.epilepsyfoundation.org/aboutepilepy/treatment/ketogenicdiet/index.cfm?gclid

Esselstyn, R. (2009). *Engine 2 diet*. New York, New York: Grand Central Life & Style.

Evans, V. (2010, November 8). Study finds exercise increases life expectancy, regardless of weight.

Evert, A. (2013, February 18). Iron in diet. *Medline Plus*. Retrieved from http://www.nlm.nih.gov.medlineplus/ency/article/002422.htm

Exercise & Calorie Guide. (n.d.) *Bruce Alora's Fitness Chart Series*. Bakersfield, CA.

Fad Diet.com. (n.d.) *Fad diets, fun and weight loss tips*. Retrieved fromhttp://www.faddiet.com/

Fad Diet.com. (n.d.). *This diet is gas powered*. Retrieved from http://www.faddiet.com/cabsoupdiet.html

Fad Diet.com. (n.d.). *Lemonade diet*. Retrieved from
http://www.faddiet.com/lemonadediet.html

Fad Diet.com. (n.d.). *The 1 day diet*. Retrieved from
http://www.faddiet.com/the-1-day-diet.html

Fad Diet.com. (n.d.). *3 day diet*. Retrieved from
http://www.faddiet.com/3daydiet.html

Fad diets: fact or fallacy? (n.d.). *University of Arkansas Division of Agriculture Research and Extension*. Retrieved from
http://www.uaex.edu/depts/FCS/EFNEP/Lessons/Fad_Diets/fad_diet
s_fact_fallacy.pdf

Fad diets. (n.d.). *Diet quotations*. Retrieved from
http://www.faddiet.com/dietquotations.hmtl

FDA. (1997, September 15). *FDA announces withdrawal of fenfluramine and dexfenfluramine (Fen-Phen)*.
http://www.fda.gov/Drugs/DrugSafety/PostmarketDrugSafetyInformati
onforPatientsandProviders/ucm179871.htm

FDA. (n.d.). *Labeling & nutrition › how to understand and use the nutrition facts label*. Retrieved from
http://www.fda.gov/Food/IngredientsPackagingLabeling/LabelingNutri
tion/ucm274593.htm

Fell, J. (2013, May 2). 15 snacks you eat at work that take you way too long to burn off the calories. *AskMen*. Retrieved from
http://www.thepostgame.com/blog/list/201305/15-snacks-you-eat-
work-take-you-way-too-long-burn#1

Ferris, R. (2013, June 19). Dunkin donuts' new gluten-free menu is a waste of money for most customers. *Business Insider*. Retrieved from
http://www.businessinsider.com/dunkin-donuts-gluten-free-menu-is-a-
waste-of-money-2013-6

Fetters, K.A. (2014, July 22). 14 fad diets you should absolutely never try. *Huffington Post*. Retrieved from http://www.huffingtonpost.com/

Fitday. (n.d.). *4 reasons why you should avoid fad diets.* Retrieved from http://www.fitday.com/fitness-articles/fitness/weight-loss/4-reasons-why-you-should-avoid-fad-diets.html

Fitday. (n.d.). *Taking laxatives to lose weight? 9 possible consequences.* Retrieved from http://www.fitday.com/fitness-articles/fitness/weight-loss/taking-laxatives-to-lose-weight?-9-possible-consequences.html

Fitsugar. (n.d.). Eating in these 5 places may be making you fat. *Yahoo! Shine.* Retrieved from http://shine.yahoo.com/healthy-living/eating-5-places-may-making-fat-224000139.html

Fitsugar.(2013, July 31). 5 reasons people give up on losing weight (and how to overcome them). *Yahoo! Shine.* Retrieved from http://shine.yahoo.com/health-living/Why-Cant-I-Lose-Weight-31055701

Fletcher, D. (2009, December 15). Fad diets. *TIME.* Retrieved from http://www.time.com/time/magazine/article/0,9171,1950931,00.html

Food Quotes. (n.d.). *The food is terrible, and the portions are too small.* Retrieved from http://www.searchquotes.com/search/Wedding_Food/2/

Fortanesce, V. (2009). *The anti-alzheimer's prescription.* New York, NY: Gotham Books, Penguin Group (USA) Inc.

Fotolio.com.(n.d.). Food and diet in Canada. *Livestrong.com.* Retrieved from http://www.livestrong.com/article/373398-food-and-diet-in-canada/

Fowler, B. (2012, November 21). Skinny Matthew McConaughey dishes on his shocking weight loss. *E! Online.* Retrieved from http://www.eonline.com/news/365424/skinny-matthew-mcconaughey-dishes-on-his-shocking-weight-loss

Fox, L. (2012, April 10). Silly diet myths that you still might be falling for – do you believe these? *Hive Health Media.* Retrieved from http://www.hivehealthmedia.com/silly-diet-myths-falling-these/

Foxcroft, L. (n.d.). Lord Byron: the celebrity diet icon. *BBC News*

Magazine. Retrieved from http://www.bbc.com/news/magazine-16351761

Freedhoff, Y. (2012, April 17). Food is not just fuel, and that matters to your diet. *U.S. News.* Retrieved from http://health.usnews.com/health-news/blogs/eat-run/2013/04/17/food-is-not-just-fuel-and-that-matters-for-your-diet

Freedhoff, Y. (2012, September 5). Exercise is not likely to be your ticket to the weight-loss express. *U.S. News.* Retrieved from http://news.yahoo.com/exercise-not-likely-ticket-weight-loss-express-131336354.html

Freeman, H. (2013, April 16). Gwyneth Paltrow and her crackpot diet may be laughable – but it's pure genius. *The Guardian.* Retrieved from http://www.guardian.co.uk/

Frighetto, J. (2012, January 24). Consumers show skepticism about some health claims on food packaging. *Neilson.* Retrieved from http://www.nielsen.com/us/en/pressroom/2012/fifty-nine-percent-of-consumers-around-the-world-indicate-diffic.html

Freuman, T.D. (2012, December 26). Why juice 'cleanses' don't deliver. *U.S. News.* Retrieved from http://health.usnews.com/health-news/blogs/eat-run/2012/12/26/why-juice-cleanses-dont-deliver

FTC. (2014, January 7). *Sensa and three other marketers of fad weight-loss products settle FTC charges in crackdown on deceptive advertising.* Retrieved from http://www.ftc.gov

FTC Consumer Information. (n.d.). *Weighing the claims in diet ads.* Retrieved from http://www.consumer.ftc.gov/articles/0061-weighing-claims-diet-ads

Furman, J. (2003). *Eat to live: the amazing nutrient-rich program for fast and sustained weight loss.* New York, NY: Little, Brown and Company.

Furst, J. (2013, June 27). Why are we obsessed with celebrities? Our DNA provides a clue. *The Daily Banter.* Retrieved from http://thedailybanter.com/2013/06/why-are-we-obsessed-with-celebrities-our-dna-provides-a-clue/

Garcia, T. (2015, April 22). Here's a clip of Dr. Oz's response to his critics. *PR Newser*. Retrieve from http://www.adweek.com/prnewser/heres-a-clip-of-dr-ozs-response-to-his-critics/113095

Gardner, A. (March 23). Atkins diet can raise heart risks. *ABC News*. Retrieved from http://abcnews.go.com/Health/Healthday/story?id=4509306

Garten, I. (2012). *Barefoot contessa foolproof*. New York, NY: Clarkson Potter.

Gavura, S. (n.d.). The Dr. Oz red palm oil (non-) miracle. *Science Based Medicine*. Retrieved from http://www.sciencebasedmedicine.org/index.php/the-dr-oz-red-palm-oil-non-miracle/

Go Pets America. (n.d.). *Multifunctional role of methionine essential amino acid. (n.d.)*. Retrieved from http://www.gopetsamerica.com/bio/methionine.aspx

Goldschmidt, D. (2015, April 22). Physicians to Columbia University: 'dismayed' Oz is on faculty. *CNN*. Retrieved from http://www.cnn.com/2015/04/17/health/dr-oz-columbia-letter/

Goldstein, S. (2013, June 10). German woman flaunts barely there 16-inch waist achieved by wearing a corset nonstop. *New York Daily News*. Retrieved from http://www.nydailynews.com/

Graham, J. (2014, January 18). Review: calorie counter apps MyFitnessPal vs. Lose It. *USA Today*. Retrieved from http://www.usatoday.com/

Gray, E. (2011, July 13). 10 fad diets to *never* try. *Huffington Post*. Retrieved from http://www.huffingtonpost.com/

Greenlaw, P., Harper, D & Greenlaw, D. (2012). *Why diets are failing us!* Denver, CO: Extaordinary Wellness Publishing.

Gupta, S. (n.d.). What's wrong with BMI. *Everyday Health*. Retrieved from http://www.everydayhealth.com/sanjay-gupta/whats-wrong-with-bmi.aspx

Hagan, C. (2009, December 15). Extreme diets: Life on 800 calories a day. *CNN Health*. Retrieved from http://www.cnn.com/2009/HEALTH/12/15/very.low.calorie.diets/index.html

Halken, M. (2013, May 17). The UK's hot new 5:2 diet craze hits the U.S. *Forbes*. Retrieved from http://.forbes.com

Hammond, P. (2015, January 10). The 20/20 diet by Dr. Phil McGraw (2015): food list. *Chewfo*. Retrieved from http://www.chewfo.com/diets/the-20-20-diet-by-dr-phil-mcgraw-food-list-what-to-eat-and-foods-to-avoid/

Harding, E. (2013, October 1), Half of women dieters admit using laxatives for quick-fix weight loss at least once despite knowing it's bad for their health. *Daily Mail*. Retrieved from http://www.dailymail.co.uk/femail/article-2440918/Half-women-dieters-admit-using-laxatives-quick-fix-weight-loss-despite-knowing-bad-health.html

Harmon, K. (2012, August 11). Early human meat-eaters thrived as vegetarian 'cavemen' Died out, researchers say. *HuffPost Science*. Retrieved from http://www.huffingtonpost.com/

Hasselbeck, E. (2009). *The g free diet*. New York, NY: Center Street.

Hatfield, H. (n.d.). Pros and cons of high-protein diets. *WebMD*. Retrieved from http://www.webmd.com/diet/features/pros-cons-of-high-protein-diets

Haupt, A. & Kotz, D. (2012, March 5). The dangers of Kardashian-endorsed QuickTrim. *US News*. Retrieved from http://health.usnews.com/health-news/diet-fitness/articles/2012/03/05/the-dangers-of-kardashian-endorsed-quicktrim-2

Haupt, A. (2013, January 4). Weight watchers diet. *US News*. Retrieved from http://health.usnews.com/best-diet/weight-watchers-diet

Haupt, A. (2013, February 7). Ashton Kutcher's fruitarian diet: what went wrong? *U.S. News*. Retrieved from http://health.usnews.com/health-news/articles/2013/02/07/ashton-kutchers-fruitarian-diet-what-went-wrong

HEALTH EDCO. (n.d.). *MyPyramid guide*. www.HealthEdco.com
Healthline Editorial Team. (2013, June 12). Can you exercise away your favorite high-calorie foods? *Healthline*. Retrieved from http://www.healthline.com/health/can-you-exercise-away-your-favorite-high-calorie-foods

Healthy Weight Forum. (n.d.). *The Scarsdale diet*. Retrieved from http://healthyweightforum.org/eng/diets/scarsdale-diet.asp

Heart & Stroke Foundation of Ontario. (n.d.). *Canadians trapped on weight-loss rollercoaster*. Retrieved from http://www.heartandstroke.on.ca/

Hegeman, R. (2015, March 23). Research into wheat variety for people with celiac disease gains new ground. *Huffington Post*. Retrieved from http://www.huffingtonpost.com/

Heid, M. (2013, July 9). Can probiotics help you lose weight. *ABC News*. Retrieved from http://abcnews.go.com/Health/Wellness/probiotics-lose-weight/story?id=19607875

Hellmich, N. (2012, December 2). New weight watchers 360 plan unveiled. *USA Today*. Retrieved from http://www.usatoday.com/

Hellmich, N. (2013, January 1). Shaping new diet and exercise habits: tips for success. *USA Today*. Retrieved from http://www.usatoday.com/

Hellmich, N. (2013, January 7). Fewer people say they're on a diet. *USA Today*. Retrieved from http://www.usatoday.com/

Hellmich, N. (2013, January 29). Study: Dieters who ate lunch earlier lost more weight. *USA Today*. Retrieved from http://www.usatoday.com/

Hellmich, N. (2013, March 19). A new fasting diet recommends that men eat just 600 calories two days a week, women, 500. *USA Today*. Retrieved from http://www.usatoday.com/

Hellmich, N. (2103, April 21). Double up: Diet, exercise together are key to success. *USA Today*. Retrieved from http://www.usatoday.com/

Hellmich, N. (2013, May 23). Would you rather lose $1,000 or gain 20 pounds? *USA Today*. Retrieved from http://www.usatoday.com/

Hellmich, N. (2013, June 19). Medical group recognizes obesity as a disease. *USA Today*. Retrieved from http://www.usatoday.com/

Hellmich, N. (2013, August 19). What's your metabolism personality type? *USA Today*. Retrieved from http://www.usatoday.com/

Henneman, A. (n.d.). Avoid portion distortion with MyPyramid's specific guidelines. *University of Nebraska*. Lincoln, NE.

Hensrud, D. (n.d.). Why do doctors recommend a slow rate of weight loss? What's wrong with fast weight loss? *Mayo Clinic*. Retrieved from http://www.mayoclinic.com/health/fast-weight-loss/AN01621

Hiser, E. (1999). *The other diabetes*. New York, NY: William Morrow.

Hitti, M. (2008, November). Lasting damage from fen-phen drug? *WebMD*. Retrieved from http://www.webmd.com/heart-disease/news/20081105/lasting-heart-damage-from-fen-phen

Hobbs, R., Broder, S., Pope, H. & Rowe, J. (2006). How adolescent girls interpret weight-loss advertising. *Oxford Journals*. Retrieved from http:her.oxfordjournals.org/content/21/5/719.full

Hodnik, J. (2012, November 1). Fad diets: The American way. [Web log post]. Retrieved from http://www.myfitnesspal.com/topics/show/785447-fad-diets-the-american-way

Holguin, J. (2004, May 29). Good news for Weight Watchers. *CBS News*.

Retrieved from http://www.cbsnews.com/news/good-news-for-weight-watchers/

Hollywood Diet. (n.d.). *About Hollywood miracle diet.* Retrieved from http://www.hollywooddiet.com/extra/about.php

Holmes, T.A. (2011, January 27). Losing weight with basal metabolic rate: the mifflin-st. jeor method. [Web log post]. *The Fitness Corner Blog.* Retrieved from http://doctorholmes.wordpress.com/2-11/01/27/losing-weight-with-basal-metabolic-rate-the-mifflin-st-jeor-method/

Horovitz, B. (2013, June 19). Taco Bell, Starbucks appeal to diet conscious eaters. *USA Today.* Retrieved from http://www.usatoday.com/

Huff Post Entertainment. (2012, December 7). *Anne Hathaway on starving for 'Les Mis': 'I just had to stop eating'.* Retrieved from http://www.huffingtonpost.com/

Huff Post Celebrity. (2013, June 28). Celebrity diets we'd never try. *Huffington Post.* Retrieved from http://www.huffingtonpost.com/

Huff Post Healthy Living. (2012, April 10). *Miley Cyrus: gluten-free diet is responsible for weight loss.* Retrieved from http://www.huffingtonpost.com/

IHRSA. (2013, June 17). *Health club industry overview.* Retrieved from http://www.ihrsa/about-the-industry

Ipatenco, S. (2014, June 8). The coconut diet plan. *LIVESTRONG.* Retrieved from http://www.livestrong.com/article/478461-the-coconut-diet-plan/

Jabr, F. (2013, June 3). How to really eat like a hunter-gatherer: why the paleo diet is half-baked. *Scientific American.* Retrieved from https://www.scientificamerican.com/article/why-paleo-diet-half-baked-how-hunter-gatherer-really-eat/

Jackson, K. (2008, December 19). Drinks diet destroyed our health. *The Sun.* Retrieved from http://www.thesun.co.uk

Jackson-Cannady, A. (2013, June). The world's healthiest diets. *FITNESS*

Magazine. Retrieved from http://shine.yahoo.com/healthy-living/worlds-healthiest-diets-142900696.html

Jarvis, S. (2014, January 27). *Fad diets: the truth behind the headlines*. [Web log post]. Retrieved from http://www.patient.co.uk/blogs/sarah-says/2014/01/fad-diets-the-truth-behind-the-headlines

Jennings, A. (2010, October 21). Drunkorexia: Alcohol mixes with eating disorders. *ABC News*. Retrieved from http://abcnews.go.com/Health/drunkorexia-alcohol-mixes-eating-disorders/story?id=11936398

Jenny Craig Official Site. (n.d.). *What's jenny all about?* Retrieved from http://www.jennycraig.com/

Johns Hopkins Health Alerts. (n.d.) Say no to high-protein diets. *Diabetes Focus*. Winter 2014. HealthCentral.com

Johnson, J.B. & Laub, Sr., D.R. (2008). *The alternate-day diet*. New York, New York: Penguin Group (USA) Inc.

Jonas-Hain, S. (2005, August 3). "Lollipop head' starlets start fashion trend. *Fox News*. Retrieved from http://www.foxnews.com/story/2005/08/03/lollipop-head-starlets-start-fashion-trend/

Jonathon. (2013, June 1). The advantages of Intermittent fasting & your first fast. *Hive Health Media*. Retrieved from http://www.hivehealthmedia.com/the-advantages-of-intermittent-fasting-your-first-fast/

Jones, J. (2012). *Wheat belly – an analysis of selected statements and basic theses from the book*. Retrieved from http://dx.doi.org/10.1094/CFW-57-4-0177

Kaiser Permanente. (n.d.). *Living Well with Diabetes Eating to Live Well (Part 2)*. Woodland Hills, CA: Regional Health Education

Kaiser Permanente. (n.d.). *Dining out: your order, please!* Department of Nutritional Services.

Kaiser Permanente. (n.d.) *Weight management*. Health Education.

Kaiser Permanente. (1995). *Increase your iron intake*. Regional Health Education.

Kaiser Permanente. (1997). *A diet for the health of your kidneys*. SCPMG Regional Health Education.

Kaiser Permanente. (1999). *Calcium*. SCPMG Regional Health Education.

Kaiser Permanente. (2003). *Dietary guidelines to decrease the risk of heart attack (Mediterranean diet)*. SCPMG Regional Health Education.

Kaiser Permanente. (2005). *Eat well, live well: eating well for your health*. SCPMG

Regional Health Education. Kaiser Permanente. (2006). *Guidelines for weight management*. SCPMG Regional Health Education.

Kaiser Permanente. (2006). *Vegetarian meal planning*. The Permanente Medical Group.

Kaiser Permanente. (2006). *Personal action plan*. SCPMG Regional Health Education.

Kaiser Permanente. (2007). *Exercise now!* SCPMG Regional Health Education.

Kaiser Permanente. (2008). *Dietary approaches to stop hypertension (the DASH diet)*. SCPMG Regional Health Education.

Kaiser Permanente. (2009). *The Healthy Plate*. SCPMG Regional Health Education.

Kaiser Permanente. (2010). *Cultivating health. Weight management kit*. Health Education Services.

Kaiser Permanente. (2011). *Calories: are you getting more than you think?* SCPMG Regional Health Education.

Kaiser Permanente. (2012). *What's in your snack?* SCPMG Regional Health Education.

Kaiser Permanente. (2012). *Cholesterol and lifestyle: take control.* SCPMG Regional Health Education.

Karst, T. (2013, July 10). Longer life linked to greater fruit and vegetable consumption. *The Packer.* Retrieved from http://www.thepacker.com/fruit-vegetable-news/Longer-life-linked-to-greater-fruit-and-vegetable-consumption-214947961.html

Katrandjian. O. (2012, January). Study finds 55 percent of nurses are overweight or obese. *ABC News.* http://abcnews.go.com/Health/study-finds-55-percent-nurses-overweight-obese/story?id=15472375

Katz, D.L. (2013, August 19). Our titanic obesity problem. *U.S. News.* Retrieved from http://news.yahoo.com/titanic-obesity-problem-211243035.html.

Kciaston. (2013, February). Coconut oil – hero or villain? *Chicago Dietetic Association.* Retrieved from http://chicagodieteticassociation.org/coconut-oil-hero-or-villain/

Kellow, J. (n.d.). Meal replacements under the spotlight. *Medifast.* Retrieved from http://www.weightlossresources.co.uk/diet/meal_replacement.htm

Kellow, J. (n.d.). *Tony Ferguson diet review.* Retrieved from http://www.weightlossresources.co.uk/diet/reviews/tony-ferguson.htm

Ketogenic Diet. (n.d.). *diabetes.co.uk.* Retrieved from http://www.diabetes.co.uk/diet/ketogenic-diet.html

Kirk, V. (n.d.). How much does nutrisystem cost in 2015? [Web log post]. *Best Diet Tips.* Retrieved from http://www.bestdiettips.com/nutritsytem/how-much-does-nutrisystem-cost-in-2011

Kirk, V. (n.d.). How much does jenny craig cost in 2015? [Web log post].

Best Diet Tips. Retrieved from http://www.bestdiettips.com/jenny-craig/how-much-does-jenny-craig-cost-price-list-for-2011

Koch, M. (2012). *Eat more of what you love.* Philadelphia, PA: Running Press.

Kopman, J. (2013, August 16). Obesity death toll heavier than previously thought. *The Weather Channel.* Retrieved from http://www.weather.com/health/obesity-death-toll-heavier-previously-thought-20130816

Kornowski, L. (2013, March 9). Gwyneth Paltrow's 'elimination diet' is hardly the craziest diet to come out of hollywood. *Huffington Post.* Retrieved from http://www.huffingtonpost.com/

Kuzemchak, S. (n.d.). The anti-diet: how not dieting is the key to losing weight. *FITNESS Magazine.* Retrieved from http://shine.yahoo.com

Lagorio, C. (2005, January 3). Diet plan success tough to weigh. *CBS News.* Retrieved from http://www.cbsnews.com/news/diet-plan-success-tough-to-weight/

Langdon, D., Reilly, P and Smilgis, M. (1980, March 31). The killing of Scarsdale diet doctor Herman Tarnower leaves a single haunting question. Why? *People.* Retrieved from http://www.people/archive/article/0,,20076135,00.html

Langley, S. (n.d.). What is naturopathy? *College of Naturopathic Medicine.* Retrieved from http://www.naturopathy-uk.com/home/home-what-is-naturopathy/

Learning ZoneExpress. (n.d.). *Think your drink.* www.learningzoneexpress.com

Learning ZoneExpress. (n.d.). *Simple Carbohydrates.* www.learningzoneexpress.com

Learning ZoneExpress. (n.d.). *Busting the myths about protein.* www.learningzoneexpress.com

Learning ZoneExpress (n.d.). *Busting the myths about vitamins.*

www.learningzoneexpress.com

Learning ZoneExpress. (n.d.). *Whole grains.* www.learningzoneexpress.com

Learning ZoneExpress. (n.d.). *Breakfast basics.* www.learningzoneexpress.com

Learning ZoneExpress. (n.d.). *Diet myths.* www.learningzoneexpress.com

Learning ZoneExpress. (n.d.). *10 ways to drink water.* www.learningzoneexpress.com

Learning ZoneExpress. (n.d.). *Portion distortion.* www.learningzoneexpress.com

Lee, E. (n.d.). The truth about red meat. *WebMD.* Retrieved from http://www.webmd.com/food-recipes/features/the-truth-about-red-meat

Lee, K. (n.d.). The slim-fast plan. *Everyday Health.* Retrieved from http://www.everydayhealth.com/diet-nutrition/the-slim-fast-plan.aspx

Leys, T. (2013, August 16). Iowa woman swallows tapeworm to lose weight. *USA Today.* Retrieved from http://www.usatoday.com/

Lillien, L. (2012). *Hungry girl to the max!* New York, NY: St. Martin's Griffin.

Lindora Clinic. (n.d.). *You have questions – we have answers.* Retrieved from http://www.lindora.com/faqs.aspx?faqID=226

London, B. (2013, May 17). The m plan: mushroom-rich diet followed by Katy Perry,

Kelly Osbourne and Roxanne Pallet can help women lose weight without shrinking their bust. *Daily Mail.* Retrieved from http://www.dailymail.co.uk/

Lynch, T.W. (2014, July 1). Pretty food really does taste better – It's Science. *Reviewed.com.*

Retrieved from http://ovens.reviewed.com/news/study-confirms-pretty-food-really-does-taste-better

Mail Online. (n.d.). Health risks of the fad diets. Retrieved from http:/www.dailymail.co.uk/health/article-129454/Health-risks-fad-diets.hmtl

Marturana, A. (n.d.) New study: why you should follow a Nordic diet. *YouBeauty.com* Retrieved from http://shine.yahoo.com/healthy-living/study-why-nordic-diet-132500989.html

Marx, R.F. (2013). Ashton Kutcher hospitalized while preparing to play Steve Jobs. *Yahoo! Movies.* https://www.yahoo.com/movies/bp/ashton-kutcher-hospitalized-while-preparing-play-steve-jobs-191433220.html

Mayo Clinic. (n.d.). *Folate.* Retrieved from http://www.mayoclinic.com/health/folate/NS_patient-folate

Mayo Clinic. (n.d.). *Thiamin (vitamin B1).* Retrieved from http://www.mayoclinic.com/health/vitamins-b1/NS_patient-thiamin

Mayo Clinic. (n.d.). *Colon cleansing: is it helpful or harmful?* Retrieved fromhttp://www.mayoclinic.com/health/colon-cleansing/AN00065

Mayo Clinic Staff. (n.d.). Calcium and calcium supplements: achieving the right balance. *Mayo Clinic.* Retrieved from http://www.mayoclinic.com/health/calcium-supplements/MY01540

Mayo Clinic Staff. (n.d.). Over-the-counter weight-loss pills: do they work? *Mayo Clinic.* Retrieved from http://www.mayoclinic.com/health/weight-loss/HQ01160

Mayo Clinic Staff. (n.d.). Prescription weight-loss drugs: can they help you? *Mayo Clinic.* Retrieved from http://www.mayoclinic.org/healthy-lifestyle/weight-loss/in-depth/weight-loss-drugs/art-20044832

Mayo Clinic Staff. (n.d.). Over-the-counter weight-loss pills: do they work? *Mayo Clinic.* Retrieved from http://www.mayoclinic.org/healthy-lifestyle/weight-loss/in-depth/weight-loss/art-20046409

Mayo Clinic Staff. (n.d.). Dash diet: healthy eating to lower your blood pressure. *Mayo Clinic.* Retrieved from http://www.mayoclinic.org/healthy-lifestyle/nutrition-and-healthy-eating/in-depth/dash/art-20048456

Mayo Clinic Staff. (n.d.). Gluten-free diet: what's allowed, what's not. *Mayo Clinic.* Retrieved from http://www.mayoclinic.com/health/gluten-free-diet/my01140

Mayo Clinic Staff. (n.d.). Low-carb diet: can it help you lose weight. *Mayo Clinic.* Retrieved from http://www.mayoclinic.com/health/low-carb-diet/nu00279/nsectiongroup=2

Mayo Clinic Staff. (n.d.) Atkins diet: What's behind the claims? *Mayo Clinic.* Retrieved from http://www.mayoclinic.com/health/atkins-diet/my00648

Mayo Clinic Staff. (n.d.). High cholesterol. *Mayo Clinic.* Retrieved from http://www.mayoclinic.com/health/niacin/CL00036

Mayo Clinic Staff. (n.d.). Alli weight-loss pill: does it work? *Mayo Clinic.* Retrieved from http://www.mayoclinic.com/health/alli/WT00030

Mayo Clinic Staff. (n.d.). South beach diet. *Mayo Clinic.* Retrieved from http://www.mayoclinic.com/health/south-beach-diet/MY00499

Mayo Clinic Staff. (n.d.). Metabolic syndrome. *Mayo Clinic.* Retrieved from http://www.mayoclinic.org/diseases/metabolic-syndrome/basics/definition/con-20027243

Mayo Clinic Staff. (2011). Exercise for weight loss: Calories burned in 1 hour. *Mayo Clinic.* Retrieved from http://www.mayoclinic.com/health/exercise/SM00109

Mayo Clinic Staff. (2011, August). Nutrition and healthy eating: glycemic index. *Mayo Clinic.* Retrieved from http://www.mayoclinic.com/health/glycemic-index-diet/MY00770

Mayo Clinic Staff. (2013). Dehydration. *Mayo Clinic.* Retrieved from http://www.mayoclinic.com/health/dehydration/DS00561/DSECTION

=complications

Mayo Clinic Staff. (2014, February 12). Food allergy. *Mayo Clinic*. Retrieved from http://www.dailymail.co.uk/femail/article-2319913/The-gluten-free-Costly-wheat-free-products-just-make-people-FATTER-health-benefits-all.html

Mayo Foundation for Medical Education and Research. (2011). *Achieving a healthy weight*. Rochester, MN.

McCaffrey, D. (2012). *The science of skinny*. Boston, MA: Lifelong Books.

McCormack, S. (2015, April, 21). Woman dies after 'dangerous' diet pills 'burn her up from within.' *The Huffington Post*. Retrieved from http://www.huffingtonpost.com

McDougall, J.A.& McDougall, M. (1995). *The McDougall program for maximum weight loss*. New York, NY: A Plume Book, Penguin Group.

McDougall, J.A. & McDougall, M. (2012). *The starch solution*. New York, NY: Rodale, Inc.

McGraw, P. (2015). *The 20/20 diet: turn your weight loss vision into reality*. Los Angeles, CA: Bird Street Books.

McMillen, M. (n.d.). Hydroxycut. *WebMD*. Retrieved from http://www.webmd.com/diet/obesity/hydroxycitric-acid-hydroxycut

Medical Dictionary. (n.d.). *Low calorie diet*. Retrieved from http://medical-dictionary. Thefreedictionary.com/low+calorie+diet

Medical News Today. (2009, May 12). *What are the eight most popular diets today?* Retrieved from http://www.medicalnwstoday.com/printerfriendlynews.php?newsid=5847

Medical News Today. (2010, March 2). *What is ketosis? What causes ketosis?* Retrieved from http://www.medicalnewstoday.com/articles/180858.php

Medifast. (n.d.). Medifast: for a slimmer, healthier you. Lose weight with

six meals a day! Retrieved from
www://www.medifast1.com/weight_loss_plan/index.jsp

Medline Plus. (n.d.). *Vitamin A*. Retrieved from
http://www.nlm.nig.gov/melineplus/ency/article/002400.htm

Men's Health. (n.d.) *20 worst drinks in America*. Retrieved from
http://eathtis.menshealth.com/slideshow/print-list/184612

Merriam-Webster. (n.d.). *yo-yo dieting*. Retrieved from
http://www.merriam-webster.com/medical/yo-yo%W20dieting.

Metcalf, E. & Zelman, K.M. (2103, November 29). Atkins diet. *WebMD*.
Retrieved from http://www.webmd.com/diet/atkins-diet-what-it-is

Michaels, J. & van Aalst, M. (2009). *Master your metabolism*. New York, NY:
Empowered Media, LLC.

MiracleGarciniaCambogia.com. (n.d.). *Stores struggle to keep the popular fat
burner in stock. Doctors call garcinia cambogia "top fat burner in a bottle."*
Retrieved from http://miraclegarciniacambogia.com/article/gs/

Mitchell, C. (2013, July 11). Fad diets: why fad is bad. *Ladue News*.
Retrieved from http://www.laduenews.com/living/health-wellness/fad-
diets-why-fad-is-bad/article_22d37955-534f-58c4-b3d8-
39e5ed9c655c.html

Miller, B. (2009, June 22). How crash diets, like the master cleanse, harm
your health and heart. *Health*. Retrieved from
http://www.health.com/health/article/0,,20409933,0.html

Moisse, K. (n.d.). Coroner links mom's death to coke 'addiction.' [Web
Log Post]. *ABC News*. Retrieved from
http://news.yahoo.com/blogs/abc-blogs/moms-death-linked-coke-
coroners-report-164723213--abc-news-health.html

Molaison, E. (2002), Stages of change in clinical nutrition practice.
Nutrition in Clinical Care, 5(5), 251-257

Moores, S. (2007, May 18). Expert warn of detox diet dangers. *NBC News*. Retrieved from http://nbcnews.com

MSN. (n.d.). *Cavemen probably had better teeth than you do, scientists say*. Retrieved from http://now.msn.com/

Murray, P.N. (2013, February 26). How emotions influence what we buy. *Psychology Today*. Retrieved from https://www.psychologytoday.com/blog/inside-the-consumer-mind/201302/how-emotions-influence-what-we-buy

Narins, E. (2013, July 3). Which impacts your weight more: diet or exercise? *Yahoo! Health*. Retrieved from http://health.yahoo.net/articles/fitness/which-impacts-your-weight-more-diet-or-exercise

Neal, H. (n.d.) New study shows dieting can actually increase unhealthy cravings. *Babble.com/Healthy Living*. Retrieved from https://ca.shine.yahoo.com/blogs/healthy-living/study-shows-dieting-actually-increase-unhealthy-cravings-221300279.html

NCES, Inch. (n.d.). *Beverages 101*.

NDEP. (n.d.). *The facts about diabetes*. Retrieved from http://ndep.nih.gov/diabetes-facts/

NEDA. (n.d.). *Effects of Media*. Retrieved from https://www.nationaleatingdisorders.org/media-body-image-and-eating-disorders

Nelson, J.K. (n.d.). What is the Special K diet? Can it help me lose weight? *Mayo Clinic*.

Retrieved from http://www.mayoclinic.com/health/special_k_diet/AN02094

Nelson, J.K. (n.d.). Does the HCG diet work – and is it safe? *Mayo Clinic*. Retrieved from http://www.mayoclinic.com/health/hcg_diet/AN02091

Neporent, L. (2011, April). Fat weight loss experts fight misperceptions.

ABC News. Retrieved from http://abcnews.go.com/Health/Diet/fat-weight-loss-experts-respect/story?id=13348969

Neporent, L. (2013, November 21). Dangerous diet trend: the cotton ball diet. *ABC News*. Retrieved from http://abcnews.go.com/Health/dangerous-diet-trend-cotton-ball-diet/story?id=20942888

Nestle, M. (2006). *What to eat*. New York, NY: North Point Press.

NewsMax. (2010, September 21). *Top five health benefits of iron*. Retrieved from http://www.newsmax.com/FastFeatures/Healthbenefitsofiron/2010/09/21/id/371069

News Medical. (2009, October 14). *Advertisements can affect women's eating behaviors and intentions to diet and exercise*. Retrieved from http://www.news-medical.net/news/20091014/Advertisements-can-affect-womens-eating-behaviors-and-intentions-to-diet-and-exercise.aspx

NHS Choices. (2011, December 9). *How to diet*. Retrieved from http://www.nhs.uk/livewell/loseweight/Pages/how-to-diet.aspx

NHS Choices. (2012, October 17). *Very low calorie diets*. Retrieved from http://www.nhs.uk/Livewell/loseweight/Pages/very-low-calorie-diets.aspx

NHS Choices. (2013, January 14). Does the 5:2 intermittent fasting diet work? Retrieved from http://www.nhs.uk/news/2013/01January/Pages/Does-the-5-2-intermittent-fasting-diet-work.aspx

Nolan, S. (2013, February 5). Man who drank eight litres of cola a day loses all his teeth – and he's still only 25. *Daily Mail*. Retrieved from http://www.dailymail.co.uk/

Nordqvist, C. (2013, May 1). What is vitamin D? What are the benefits of vitamin D? *Medical News Today*. Retrieved from http://www.medicalnewstoday.com/

Nordqvist, C. (2013, November 26). What is the vegetarian diet? What are the benefits of a vegetarian diet? *Medical News Today*. Retrieved from http://www.medicalnewstoday.com/articles/8749.php

Novak, S. (2011, December 20). What did cavemen really eat and were they actually healthier? [Web log post]. *Discovery*. Retrieved from http://blogs.discovery.com/dfh-sara-novak/2011/12/what-did-cavemen-really-eat-and-were-they-actually-healthier.html

Nutrisystem. (n.d.). *How nutrisystem works*. Retrieved from http://www.nutrisystem.com/

Nutrition Action Newsletter. (2008). *Can you afford the extras?* Med. Sci. Sports Exerc. 32:S498, 2000. Nutritionallyfit. (2013, March, 15). *Wheat belly diet? The skinny on wheat in your diet*. Retrieved from http://nutritionally-fit.com/nutrition/wheat-belly-diet

O'Malley, M. (2015, January 27). *Dr. Oz's favorite weight loss pill is a hoax, government says*. Retrieved from http://www.everydayhealth.com/columns/daily-checkup/green-coffee-bean-extract-dr-oz-diet-secret-weapon-disarmed-by-ftc/

Office of Dietary Supplements, National Institutes of Health. (n.d.). *Vitamin A*. Retrieved from http://ods.od.nih.gov/factsheets/VitaminA-QuickFacts/

Office of Dietary Supplements, National Institutes of Health. (n.d.). *Vitamin C*. Retrieved from http://ods.od.nih.gov/factssheets/VitaminC-HealthProfessional/

Office of Dietary Supplements, National Institutes of Health. (2011). *Vitamin B6*. Retrieved from http://ods.od.nih.gov/factsheets/VitaminB6-QuickFacts/

Ogilvie, J.P. (2012, June 9). Dietary cleanses rise in popularity, but there are risks. *Los Angeles Times*. Retrieved from http://articles.latimes.com/

Oldenburg, A. (2013, April 9). Trisha Yearwood wows with weight loss. *USA Today*. Retrieved from http://www.usatoday.com/

Orelli, B. (2013, November 30). The best obesity drug is yet to come. *The Motley Fool.* Retrieved from http://www.fool.com/investing/general/2013/11/30/arena-and-vivus-emerging-competitor.aspx

OMG Facts. (October 28) *In 1974, a British health nut drank himself to death with carrot juice.* Retrieved from http://www.omgfacts.com/lists/4882/In-1974-a-British-health-nut-drank-himself-to-death-with-carrot-juice

Ornish, D. (2000). *Dean Ornish's program for reversing heart disease.* New York, NY: The Random House Publishing Group.

Ornish, D. (2007). *The spectrum.* New York, NY: Ballantine Books.

Orr, T. (2010, October 12). Fad diets: fad dieting failures reveal Americans attitudes toward food and themselves. *Pacific Standard.* Retrieved from http://www.psmag.com/health-and-behavior/fad-diets-a-losing-battle-23918

Painter, K. (2014, February 27). Proposed food labels stress calories, sugar, portions. *USA Today.* Retrieved from http://www.usatoday.com/

Paleo Diet. (n.d.). *The primary characteristics of the paleo diet.* Retrieved from http://thepaleodiet.com/the-paleo-diet-premise/

Paltrow, G. & Turshen, J. (2013). *It's all good.* New York, NY: Grand Central Life & Style.

Paris, C.B. (2015, March 17). France moves to outlaw skinny models. *The Times.* Retrieved from http://www.thetimes.co.uk/tto/world/europe/article4384124.ece

Park, A. (n.d.). Tube feeding: what's wrong with the latest wedding crash diet? *TIME.* Retrieved from http://healthlandtime.com/2012/04/18/with-this-tube-i-thee-shed-whats-wrong-with-the-latest-wedding-crash-diet/

Park, A. (2011, July 20). Are calorie counts on menus accurate? Not so much. *TIME.* Retrieved from http://healthland.time.com/2011/07/20/are-calorie-counts-on-menus-accurate-not-so-much/

Patton, L. (n.d.). Dunkin' to sell gluten-free doughnuts in fast-food first. *Yahoo! Finance*. Retrieved from http://finance.yahoo.com/news/dunkin-sell-gluten-free-doughnuts-201603674.html

Pavini, J. (2013, May 14). Weight-loss scams lighten only your wallet. *Jeanette Pavini's Buyer Beware*. Retrieved from http://www.marketwatch.com

Perrone, M. (2014, January 8). FTC cracks down on weight-loss products. *The Boston Globe*. Retrieved from http://www.bostonglobe.com/

Phillips, T. (2007, January 13). Anna Carolina Reston: the model who starved herself to death. *The Guardian*. Retrieved from http://www.theguardian.com/

Physicians Committee for Responsible Medicine. (n.d.). *The protein myth*. Retrieved from http://www.pcrm.org/healthy/diets/vsk/vegetarian-starter-kit-protein

Picco, M.F. (n.d.). Is colon cleansing a good way to eliminate toxins from your body? *Mayo Clinic*. Retrieved from http://www.mayoclinic.com/health/colon-cleansing/AN00065

Poladian, C. (2013, January 3). Red palm oil, latest diet miracle promoted by Dr. Oz. does it work? *International Business Times*. Retrieved from http://www.cleanprogram.com/media/files/clean-program-manual.pdf

Pollan, M. (2009). *Food rules an eater's manual*. New York, NY: Penguin Books.

Poortmans, J.R. & Dellalieux, O. (2000, March). Do regular high protein diets have potential health risks on kidney function in athletes. *Int J Sport Nutr Exerc Metab*. 10(1):28-38. Retrieved from http://www.ncbi.nlm.nih.gov/pubmed/10722770

Power, M. (2013, May 9). The gluten free con: It's the stars' favourite food fad. But costly wheat-free products just make most people fatter –

with no benefits at all. *Mail Online*. Retrieved from
http://www.dailymail.co.uk/

Preidt, R. (2013, March 6). Steer clear of 'miracle cure,' other bogus health
products. *Everyday Health*. Retrieved from
http://consumer.healthday.com/public-health-information-30/food-and-
drug-administration-news-315/steer-clear-of-miracle-cures-other-bogus-
health-products-fda-674100.html

Prigg, M. (n.d.). Official: Atkins is a health risk. *Daily Mail*. Retrieved from
http://www.dailymail.co.uk/

Radar Online. (2013, September 17). *Lawsuit evaporates…just like the weight!*
Kardashian sisters score major victory in $5m "quick trim" class action. Retrieved
from http://radaronline.com/exclusives/2013/09/kardashian-quick-trim-
lawsuit-dismissed/

Rainbird, A. (2013, April 26). Mathew McConaughey: how I slimmed
down to 9.5 stone for "incredible" film role. *Mirror*. Retrieved from
http://www.mirror.co.uk/

Ratey, J.J. & Hagerman, E. (2008). *Spark*. New York, NY: Little, Brown
and Company.

Ravitz, J. (2013, March). Gwyneth Paltrow makes kids avoid carbs: Apple,
Moses are often hungry. *Us Magazine*. Retrieved from
http://www.usmagazine.com/celebrity-body/news/gwyneth-paltrow-
makes-kids-avoid-carbs-apple-moses-are-often-hungry-2013133

Reaney, P. (2015, January 6). DASH named best overall diet for fifth year:
report. *Reuters*. Retrieved from
http://www.reuters.com/article/2015/01/06/health-diets-
idUSL1N0UK21V20150106

Redfern, C. (2012, December 26). "I was a witch. It's a miracle my
relationship survived": Anne Hathaway talks about dieting for Les
Miserables. *Mirror*. Retrieved from
http://www.mirror.co.uk/3am/celebrity-news/anne-hathaway-tells-
chelsea-handler-1506317

Reinagel, M. (2013, January 2). Color confusion: identifying red meat and white meat. *Food & Nutrition Magazine*. Retrieved from http://www.foodandnutrition.org/

Reisner, R. (2008). The diet industry: a big fat lie. *Business Week*. Retrieved from http://www.businessweek.com/debateroom/archives/2008/03/the_diet _industry_a_big_fat_lie

Relaxnews. (2013, November 25). Five worst celebrity diets to avoid in the new year. *Yahoo News*. Retrieved from http://news.yahoo.com/five-worst-celebrity-diets-avoid-112644538.html

Reno, C. (2009). *The eat-clean diet recharged*. Mississauga, ON Canada: Robert Kennedy Publishing.

Rettner, R. (n.d.). Woman drinks only soda for 16 years, suffers heart problems. *LiveScience.com*. Retrieved from http://news.yahoo.com/woman-drinks-only-soda-16-years-suffers-heart-111020462.html

Rettner, R. & My Health Daily. (2013, March 11). Most people shouldn't eat gluten free. *Scientific American*. Retrieved from http://www.scientificamerican.com/article.cfm?id=most-people-shouldn't-eat-gluten-free

Rettner, R. (2013, September 8). M plan, new mushroom diet promising selective weight loss, won't work, experts say. *The Huffington Post*. Retrieved from http://www.huffingtonpost.com./

Riggle, A. (2012, January 31). Fad diets lead to weight loss failure. *Daily Sundial*. Retrieved from http://sundial.csun.edu/2012/01/fad-diets-lead-to-weight-loss-failure/

Robinson, J. (2013). *Eating on the wild side*. New York, NY: Little, Brown and Company.

Rolls, B & Harmann, M. (2012). *The ultimate volumetrics diet*. New York, NY: William Morrow.

Rosen, M. (1994, January 10). Oprah overcomes. *People Magazine.* Retrieved from http://www.people.com/people/archive/article/0,,20107260,00.html

Rotchford, L.(n.d.). *Diets through history: the good, bad and scary.* Retrieved from http://www.health.com/health/gallery/0,,20653382_3,00.html

Rothman, J. (n.d.). Does the master cleanse work? *Everyday Health.* Retrieved from http://www.everydayhealth.com/weight/does-the-master-cleanse-work.aspx

Saad, L. (2013). To lose weight, Americans rely more on dieting than exercise. *Gallup, Inc.* Retrieved from http://www.gallup.com/poll/150986/Lose-Weight-Americans-Rely-Dieting-Exercise.aspx

Saguy, A. (2013, January 4). Why we diet. *Los Angeles Times.* Retrieved from http://articles.latimes.com/

Sakimura, J. (2013, July 10). Coconut oil: the good, the bad, and the unknown. *Everyday Health.* Retrieved from http://www.everydayhealth.com/columns/johannah-sakimura-nutrition-sleuth/coconut-oil-the-good-the-bad-and-the-unknown/

Sanfilippo, D. (2012). *Practical paleo.* Las Vegas, NV: Victory Belt Publishing, Inc.

Singal, J. (2015, March 18). Watching cooking shows might lead to weight gain. *Science of Us.* Retrieved from http://nymag.com/scienceofus/2015/03/cooking-shows-might-lead-to-weight-gain.html

Sass, C. (2013, January 22). Pros and cons of the alkaline diet. *Fox News.* Retrieved from http://www.foxnews.com/health/2013/01/21/pros-and-cons-alkaline-diet/

Sass, C. (2013, January 31). Ashton Kutcher's diet scare: 5 fad-diet red flags. *Fox News Magazine.* Retrieved from http://magazine.foxnews.com/food-wellness/ashton-kutchers-diet-scare-

5-fad-diet-red-flags

Satherly, J. (2010, March 23). Dave Grohl rushed to hospital after coffee overdose. *Metro News*. Retrieved from http://metro.co.uk/2010/03/23/dave-grohl-rushed-to-hospital-after-coffee-overdose-187627/

Science Daily. (2010, January 9). *Study examines calorie information from restaurants, packaged foods*. Retrieved from http://www.sciencedaily.com/releases/2010/01/100106095051.htm

Science Daily. (2013, May 13). *Individual and small-chain restaurant meals exceed recommended daily calorie needs*. Retrieved from http://www.sciencedaily.com/releases/2013/05/130513174005.htm

Scott, J.R. (2009, May 13). An overview of the Atkins diet. *About.com*. Retrieved from http://weightloss.about.com/od/theatkinsdiet/a/atkinsoverview.htm

Sepkowitz, K. (n.d.). Introducing 'breatharianism,' the dumbest diet of all time. *The Daily Beast*. Retrieved from http://www.thedailybeast.com/articles/2014/03/02/introducing-breatharianism-the-dumbest-diet-of-all-time.html

Shapiro, H.M. (2001). *Picture perfect weight loss shopper's guide*. New York, NY: Rodale, Inc.

Shapiro, H.M. & Becker, F. (2010). *Eat & beat diabetes with picture perfect weight loss*. Ontario, Canada: Harlequin Enterprises Limited.

Shepard, S. (2013, May 30). Is eating too much wheat bad for your health? *Fact Buster*. Retrieved from http://www.abc.net.au/health/talkinghealth/factbuster/stories/2013/05/30/3770812.htm

Shenker, M. (2011, June 2). Sugar busters' diet menus. *Livestrong.com*. Retrieved from http://www.livestrong.com/article/461172-sugar-busters-diet-menus/

Shenker, M. (2011, July 24). Side effects of the Hollywood 48 hour miracle diet. *LiveStrong*. Retrieved from http://www.livestrong.com/article/500277-side-effects-of-the-hollywood-48-hour-miracle-diet/

Singal, J. (2015, March 18). Watching cooking shows might lead to weight gain. *Science of Us*. Retrieved from http://nymag.com/scienceofus/2015/03/cooking-shows-might-lead-to-weight-gain.html

Sisson, M. (2012). *The primal blueprint*. Malibu, CA: Primal Nutrition, Inc.

Smith, J. (2012, September 28). How (in)accurate are calorie counters at the gym? *Shape*. Retrieved from http://www.shape.com/fitness/cardio/how-inaccurate-are-calorie-counters-gym

Smith, J. (2013, May 30). 10 reasons why cavemen were healthier than modern man. *Toronto Examiner*. Retrieved from http://www.examiner.com/

Smith, I.K. (n.d.). *SHRED the revolutionary diet*. Retrieved from http://www.doctoriansmith.com/books/shred-the-revolutionary-diet/

Sole, E. (2013, April 8). The paleo diet, debunked. *Yahoo! Shine*. Retrieved from http://shine.yahoo.com/healthy-living/the-paleo-diet-debunked

South Beach Diet. (n.d.). *Overview of the south beach diet gluten solution program*. Retrieved from http://southbeachdiet.com/diet/south-beach-diet-gluten-solution-program

Spano, M. (n.d.). Paleo diet: pros and cons. *Cooking Light*. Retrieved from http://www.cookinglight.com/eating-smart/nutrition-101/paleo-diet-00412000080115/

Spector, D. (2013, February). 25-year-old soda addict loses all his teeth. *Mandatory Newsletter*. Retrieved from http://www.mandatory.com/2013/02/11/25-year-old-soda-addict-loses-all-his-teeth/

Starbucks Coffee Company. (2010). *Nutrition by the cup.*

Starbucks Coffee Company. (2013). *Food Facts.*

Stein, J. (2010, January 10), Hours sitting in front of TV found to shorten life. *Los Angeles Times.* Retrieved from http://articles.latimes.com

Steinberg, D.M., Bennett, G.G., Askew, S. & Tate, D.F. (2015, February 12). Weighing every day matters: daily weighing improves weight loss and adoption of weight control behaviors. *Journal of the Academy of Nutrition and Dietetics.* 115(4).

Stobe, M. (2013, July 22). Skipping breakfast may increase heart attack risk. *Yahoo! News.* Retrieved from http://news.yahoo.com/skipping-breakfast-may-increase-heart-attack-risk-210037837.html

Strawbrideg, H. (2013, February 20). Going gluten-free just because? Here's what you need to know. [Web log post]. *Harvard Health Publications.* Retrieved from

http://www.health.harvard.edu/blog/going-gluten-free-just-because-heres-what-you-need-to-know-201302205916

Strong, D. (2013, December 30). The 10 most famous diets of all time. *Everyday Health.* Retrieved from http://www.everydayhealth.com/food/the-10-most-famous-fad-diets-of-all-time.aspx

Stylist Staff. (2014, September 26). *Do men and women react differently to a fat first date?* Retrieved from http://www.stylist.com/read/do-men-and-women-react-differently-to-a-fat-first-date/

Surrell, J.A. (2011). *SOS diet.* Newberry, Michigan: Bean Books, LLC.

Sweetwaterhrv. (2012, April 6). *Heart disease plagued cavemen, too.* [Web log post]. Retrieved from http://sweetwaterhrv.com/blog/heart-rate-variability/heart-disease-plagued-cavemen-too/

Szabo, L. (2013, January 18). Book raises alarms about alternative medicine. *USA Today.* Retrieved from http://www.usatoday.com/

Taboola. (2013, April 23). Kelly Osbourne's weight loss is hard to maintain: "you have to commit to a life change.' *HuffPost Celebrity*. Retrieved from http://www.huffingtonpost.com

Tauber, M & Williams, A. (n.d.). Extreme measures. *People Magazine*. Retrieved from http://www.people.com/people/archive/0.20060671,00.html

The Cleveland Clinic Foundation. (2012). *Stay fit*. Retrieved from http://myclevelandclinic.org/healthy_living/weight_control/hic_fad_diet s.aspx

The Daily Meal. (2013, August 3). *Diets that don't work*. Retrieved from http://shine.yahoo.com/healthy-living/diets-dont-205000297.html

The Huffington Post. (2013, February 12). *Natasha Harris died from drinking too much coke, New Zealand coroner says*. Retrieved from http://huffingtonpost.com/

The Huffington Post. (2013, November 26). *How Kelly Osbourne dropped 70 pounds, and kept the weight off*. Retrieved from http://huffingtonpost.com/

The Huffington Post. (2014, June 12). *Why diet and exercise are not the keys to weight loss and health*. Retrieved from http://huffingtonpost.com/

The Huffington Post Canada. (2014, May 14). *Gluten intolerance may be completely fake:study*. Retrieved from http:huffingtonpost.ca/

The Primary Characteristics of the Paleo Diet. (n.d.). Retrieved from http://thepaleodiet/com/the-paleo-diet-premise/

The Right Chef – Immuno Laboratories, Inc. (n.d.) Rating the sugar busters diet: advantages and disadvantages. *BetterHealthUSA*. Retrieved from http://www.betterhealthusa.com/public/252.cfm

The Week's Editorial Staff. (2013, April 7). Is going gluten-free healthier for everybody? *Yahoo*. http://news.yahoo.com/going-gluten-free-healthier-everybody-090000239.html

The Weight Loss Experts at Mayo Clinic. (2010). *The mayo clinic diet.* Intercourse, PA: Good Books.

The World's Healthiest Foods. (2015, December 9). *Mushrooms, crimini.* Retrieved from http://www.whfoods.com/genpage.php?tname=foodspice&dbid=9 7

Thompson, D. (2015, January 6). Diet rich in whole grains might extend your life. *HealthDay News.* Retrieved from http://consumer.healthday.com/senior-citizen-information-31/misc-aging-news-10/diet-rich-in-whole-grains-might-extend-your-life-study-says-695204.html

TVTopTen.com (n.d.). *Jenny Craig vs. Nutrisystem – diet comparison.* Retrieved from http://www.tvtopten.com/jenny-craig-vs-nutrisystem.html UCLA Center for Human Nutrition. (n.d.). *Dietary programs / very low calorie diet (VLCD).*Retrieved from http://rfoweightloss.med.ucls.edu/body.cfm?id=32

University of Wisconsin School of Medicine and Public Health. (n.d.). *The reality behindgluten-free diets.* Retrieved from http://www.uwheatlh.org/nutrition-diet/the-reality-behind-gluten-free-diets/31084

USDA. (n.d.). *Choose My Plate.* Retrieved from http://www.choosemyplate.gov

USDA. (n.d.). *Food labeling.* Retrieved from http://www.choosemyplate.gov/supertracker-tools/food-labeling.html

USDA Center for Nutrition Policy and Promotion. (2011). *Build a healthy meal.*

U.S. Food and Drug Administration. (2014, November 25). *FDA finalizes menu and vending calorie labeling rules.* Retrieved from http://www.fda.gov/NewsEvents/Newsroom/PressAnnouncements/uc m423952.htm

US News. (n.d.). *Medifast*. Retrieved from http://health.usnews.com/best-diet/medifast-diet

US News. (n.d.) *Raw food diet*. Retrieved from http://health.usnews.com/best-diet/raw-food-diet

US News. (n.d.) *Nutrisystem diet*. Retrieved from http://health.usnews.com/best-diet/nutrisystem-diet/reviews

US News. (n.d.). *Weight watchers diet*. Retrieved from http://health.usnews.com/best-diet/weight-watchers-diet

US News. (n.d.). *Paleo diet*. Retrieved from http://health.usnews.com/best-diet/paleo-diet

Us Weekly. (2013). *Miss USA 2013 contestants too skinny, former pageant winners say*. Yahoo! Retrieved from http://omg.yahoo.com/news/

Us Weekly. (2015). *Kai Hibbard, the biggest loser contestant, lifts lid on shocking show secrets, claims mental and physical abuse*. Retrieved from https://celebrity.yahoo.com/news/kai-hibbard-biggest-loser-contestant-lifts-lid-shocking-131223095-us-weekly.html

Vaccariello, L. & Sass, C. (2008). *Flat belly diet!* New York, New York: Rodale, Inc.

Vann, M. (n.d.). Probiotics and weight loss. *Everyday health*. Retrieved from http://www.everydayhealth.com

Virgin, J.J. (2012). *The virgin diet*. Ontario, Canada: Harlequin.

Vitelli, R. (2009, October 8). Does food advertising affect eating habits? [Web log post] *Providentia*. Retrieved from http://drvitelli.typepad.com/providentia/2009/10/does-food-advertising-affect-eating-habits.html

Wanjek, C. (2015, June 29). Sugary drinks kill 184,000 people every year. *Live Science*. Retrieved from http://www.yahoo.com

Ward, A. (2013, May 29). Man dies from drinking too much coca-cola,

rules British coroner. *Newsmax*. Retrieved from
http://www.newmax.com/thewire/man-dies-drinking-coca-
cola/2013/05/29/id/506922

WebMD. (n.d.). *Fasting diets*. Retrieved from
http://www.webmd.com/food-recipes/guide/fasting

WebMD. (n.d.). *The truth about fad diets*. Retrieved from
http://www.webmd.boots.com/diet/guide/the-truth-about-fad-diets

WebMD. (n.d.). *The grapefruit diet plan review*. Retrieved from
http://webmd.com/diet/features/the-grapefruit-diet

WebMD. (n.d.). *Obesity, weight loss, and very low-calorie diets (VLCDs)*.
Retrieved from http://www.webmd.com/diet/low-calorie-diets

WebMD. (n.d.) *Methionine*. Retrieved from
http://www.webmd.com/vitamins-supplements/ingredientmono-42-
methionine.aspx?activeingredientid=42&activeingredientname=methionie

WebMD. (n.d.) *Losing weight without fad diets*. Retrieved from
http://www.webmd.com/diet/guide/the-truth-about-fad-diets

WebMD. (n.d.). *The biggest loser diet*. Retrieved from
http://webmd.com/diet/biggest-loser-diet?page=2

WebMD. (n.d.). *Hydroxycut*. Retrieved from
http://webmd.com/diet/hydroxycitric-acid-hydroxycut

WebMD. (n.d.) *The Jenny Craig weight loss program*. Retrieved from
http://www.webmd.com/diet/jenny-craig-what-it-is

WebMD. (n.d.). *Volumetrics*. Retrieved from
http://www.webmd.com/diet/volumetrics-what-it-is

WebMD. (n.d.). *The flat belly diet*. Retrieved from
http://www.webmd.com/diet/belly-fat-diet

WebMD. (n.d.). *Green coffee*. Retrieved from http://www.webmd.com

WebMD. (n.d.). *Palm oil*. Retrieved from http://www.webmd.com

WebMD. (n.d.). *Garcinia*. Retrieved from http://www.webmd.com

WebMD. (n.d.). *Raspberry ketone*. Retrieved from http://www.webmd.com

WebMD. (n.d.). *Copper*. Retrieved from http://www.webmd.com

WebMD. (n.d.). *Garcinia cambogia: safe for weight loss?* Retrieved from http://www.webmd.com/vitamins-and-supplements/garcinia-weight-loss?page=2

WebMD. (n.d.). *Macrobiotic diet*. Retrieved from http://www.webmd.com/diet/macrobiotic-diet

WebMD. (n.d.). *Alkaline diets*. Retrieved from http://www.webmd.com/diet/alkaline-diets

WebMD. (n.d.). *Natural colon cleansing: is it necessary?* Retrieved from http://www.webmd.com/balance/guide/natural-colon-cleansing-is-it-necessary

WebMD. (2008). *High protein, low carb diets*. Retrieved from http://www.webmd.com/diet/high-protein-low-carbohydrate-diets

WebMD. (2009). *Chromium – topic overview*. Retrieved from http://www.webmd.com/digestive-disorders/tc/chromium-topic-overview

WebMD. (2012). *Acai berries and acai berry juice – what are the health benefits?* Retrieved from http://www.webmd.com/diet/acai-berries-and-acai-berry-juice-what-are-the-health-benefits

WebMD. (2012, February 1). *Calculating your waist circumference*. Retrieved from http://www.webmdcom/diet/calculating-your-waist-circumference_

Wedner, J. (2015, March 20). Belly-busting restaurant meals. *Lifescript*. Retrieved from http://www.lifescript.com/health/centers/obesity/articles/belly-busting_restaurant_meals.aspx

Westerterp,K.R. (2004, August 18). Diet induced thermogenesis. *Nutr Metab.* (Lond). 1:5. Retrieved from http://www.ncbi.nlm.hih.gov/pmc/articles/PMC524030/

Westerterp-Plantenga, M.S. (2000, March). Satiety and 24h diet-induced thermogenesis as related to macronutrient composition. *Scand J Nutr/Naringsforskning.* Retrieved from http://www.foodandnutritionresearch.net/index.php/fnr/article/view/1 777

Westman, E.C., Phinney, S.D. & Volek, J.S. (2010). *The new atkins for a new you.* New York, New York: Touchstone.

White, M.C. (2013, March 13). Why we're wasting billions on gluten-free food. *TIME.* Retrieved from http://business.time.com/2013/03/13/why-were-wasting-billions-on-gluten-free-food/

White, S. (n.d.). Lemonade diet: Beyoncé's maple syrup weight loss secret. *Calorie Lab.* Retrieved from http://calorielab.com/news/2006/08/18/weight-loss-with-the-maple-syrup-diet/

WHO. (2015, January). *Diabetes.* Retrieved from http://www.who.int/mediacentre/factsheets/fs312/en/

Willet, W.C. & Skerrett, P.J. (2001). New York, NY: Free Press.

Williams, G. (2013, January 2). The heavy price of losing weight. *U.S. News.* Retrieved from http://money.usnews.com/money/personal-finance/articles/2013/01/02/the-heavy-price-of losing-weight

Williams, S. (2013, December 2). This new data shows we're on the wrong path to treating obesity. *The Motley Fool.* Retrieved from http://www.fool.com/investing/general/2013/12/02/this-new-data-shows-were-on-the-wrong-path-to-trea.aspx

Wilson, F.A., van den Borne, J.J.G.C., Calder, A.G, O'Kennedy, N., Holtrop, G., Rees, W.D., & Lobley, G.E. (2009, April 1). Tissue methionine cycle activity and homocysteine metabolism in female rats: impact of dietary methionine and folate plus choline. *American Journal of Physiology Endocrinology and Metabolism*. Retrieved from http://ajpendo.physiology.org/content/296/4/E702

Wilson, J. (2013, June 19). Physicians group labels obesity a disease. *CNN*. Retrieved from http://www.cnn.com/2013/06/19/health/ama-obesity-disease-change/

WIN. (2008, August). *Very low-calorie diets*. Retrieved from http://win.niddk.nig.gov/publications/low_calorie.htm

Winter, M. (2013, March 19). Study links 180,000 global death to sugary drinks. *USA Today*. Retrieved from http://www.usatoday.com/

Winterman, D. (2013, January 2). History's weirdest fad diets. *BBC News Magazine*. Retrieved from http://www.bbc.com/news/magazine-20695743

Woolston, C. (2012, May 19). Are raspberry ketones a 'miracle' fat burner? Dr. Oz weighs in. Retrieved from http://articles.latimes.com/

Woolston, C. (2013, October 26). Alkaline diet claims get sour response from doctors. *Los Angeles Times*. Retrieved from http://articles.latimes.com/2013/oct/26/health/la-he-1026-alkaline-20131026

Women's Health Magazine. (2012, March). Detox diet: how a juice cleanse affect your body. *Rodale, Inc.* Retrieved from http://womenshealthmag.com/weight-loss/detox-diet-side-effects

Women's Health Magazine. (2015, March). *Health scoop!* Rodale, Inc.

World Health Organization. (2013). *Obesity and overweight*. Retrieved from http://www.who.int/mediacentre/factsheets/fs311/en/

Wurtman, J.J. (2013, August 1). Juice cleanses: the new eating disorder?

HuffPost Health Living. Retrieved from http://www.huffingtonpost.com/

Yo yo dieting. (n.d.). In *Merriam-Webster's online dictionary.* Retrieved from http://www.meriam-webster.com/dictionary/yo-yodieting

Yu, C. ((2014, July 18). Waist training: can you cinch your waist thin? *The Daily Beast.* Retrieved from http://www.thedailybeast.com/articles/2014/07/18/waist-training-can-you-cinch-your-waist-thin.html

Yu, W. (2014, November 23). 10 foods overweight people eat regularly. *The Huffington Post.* Retrieved from http://www.huffingtonpost.com/

Zelman, K. (n.d.). The baby food diet: review. *WebMD.* Retrieved from http://www.webmd.com/diet/features/baby-food-diet-review?page=2

Zelman, K.M. (n.d.). The truth about sensa. *WebMD.* Retrieved from http://www.webmd.com/diet/features/truth-about-sensa

Zelman, K.M. (n.d.). The truth about hCG for weight loss. *WebMD.* Retrieved from http://www.webmd.com/diet/features/truth-about-hcg-for-weight-loss

Zelman, K.M. (n.d.). The medifast diet plan. *WebMD.* Retrieved from http://www.webmd.com/diet/features/the-medifast-diet-plan

Zelman, K.M. (n.d.). The lemonade diet (master cleanse diet). *WebMD.* Retrieved from http://www.webmd.com/diet/features/the-lemonade-diet-master-cleanse-diet

Zelman, K.M. (n.d.). The 'biggest loser' diet. *WebMD.* Retrieved from http://www.webmd.com/diet/features/biggest-loser-diet.

Zelman, K.M. (n.d.). Weight watchers points plus: diet review. *WebMD.* Retrieved from http://www.webmd.com/diet/features/weight-watchers-diet

Zelman, K.M. (n.d.). The cookie diet. *WebMD.* Retrieved from http://www.webmd.com/diet/features/the-cookie-diet

Zelman, K.M. (n.d.). Acai: Weight loss wonder fruit? *WebMD*. Retrieved from http://webmd.com/diet/features/acai-weight-loss-wonder-fruit

Zelman, K.M. (n.d.). The O2 diet. *WebMD*. Retrieved from http://www.webmd.com/diet/features/the-o2-diet

Zelman, K.M. (n.d.). The NutriSystem diet. *WebMD*. Retrieved from http://www.webmd.com/diet/features/the-nutrisystem-diet

Zelman, K.M. (n.d.). Body for Life. *WebMD*. Retrieved from http://www.webmd.com/diet/features/body_for_life_what_it_is

Zelman, K>M. & Fields, L. (n.d.). The sugar busters! diet. *WebMD*. Retrieved from http://www.webmd.com/diet/sugar-busters-what-it-is

Zelman, K.M. (2010). Diet review: The caveman (paleo) diet. *WebMD*. Retrieved from http://www.webmd.com/diet/features/diet-review-the-caveman-paleo-diet?page=2

Zelman, K.M. & Levitt, S. (2013). The zone diet. *WebMD*. Retrieved from http://www.webmd.com/diet/zone-what-it-is

Zeratsky, K. (n.d.). Are high-protein diets safe for weight loss. *Mayo Clinic*. Retrieved from http://www.mayoclinic.com/health/high-protein-diets/AN00847

Zeratsky, K. (n.d.) I'm considering having my ears stapled to help me lose weight. Does this work? *Mayo Clinic*. Retrieved from http://www.mayoclinic.com/health/ear-stapling-for-weight-loss/AN01476

Zeratsky, K. (n.d.). I'm thinking about trying a diet pill called lipovarin. Can you tell me if it really works? *Mayo Clinic*. Retrieved from http://www.mayoclinic.com/health/lipovarin/AN01489

Zeratsky, K. (n.d.). How do weight-loss products such as sense, slimscents and aroma patch work? *Mayo Clinic*. http://www.mayoclinic.com/health/sensa/AN02050

Zeratsky, K. (n.d.). Drinking apple cider vinegar for weight loss seems far-fetched. Does it work? *Mayo Clinic.* Retrieved from http://www.mayoclinic.com/health/apple-cider-vinegar-for-weight-loss/AN01816

Zeratsky, K. (n.d.). Are vitamin B-12 injections helpful for weight loss? *Mayo Clinic.* Retrieved from http://www.mayoclinic.com/health/vitamin-b12injections/AN01400

Zeratsky, K. (n.d.). Can coconut oil help me lose weight? *Mayo Clinic.* Retrieved from http://www.mayoclinic.com/health/coconut-oil-and-weight-loss/AN01899

Zeratsky, K. (n.d.). What is the cabbage soup diet, and can it help me lose weight? *Mayo Clinic.* Retrieved from http://www.mayoclinic.com/health/cabbage-soup-diet/AN02134

Zeratsky, K. (2012). Do detox diets offer any health benefits? *Mayo Clinic.* Retrieved from http://www.mayoclinic.com/health/detox-diets/AN01334

Zimney, E. (2006, December 14). Master cleanse diet = master scam. [Web log post]. Retrieved from http://www.everydayhealth.com/columns/zimney-health-and-medical-news-you-can-use/master-cleanse-diet-master-scam/

Zinczenko, D. & Goulding, M. (2009). *Eat this not that!* New York, NY: Rodale, Inc.

Zinczenko, D. & Goulding, M. (2010). *Cook this not that!* New York, NY: Rodale, Inc.

Zinczenko, D. & Goulding, M. (2011). *Eat this not that!* New York, NY: Rodale, Inc.

Zinczenko, D. & Goulding, M. (2011). *The eat this not that diet.* New York, NY: Rodale, Inc.

LISA TILLINGER JOHANSEN

The information contained in this book is intended to be used as a general guideline only. For individuals with specific questions, problems, diseases and conditions, please contact your health care provider.

LISA TILLINGER JOHANSEN

ABOUT THE AUTHOR

LISA TILLINGER JOHANSEN is a Registered Dietitian with a masters degree in nutritional science. She teaches nutrition classes and counsels patients on a wide range of health issues. Her nonfiction debut book, *Fast Food Vindication*, received the Discovery Award in the Health/Nutrition category. She lives in Southern California.

LISA TILLINGER JOHANSEN